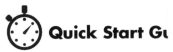

Quick Start Gu

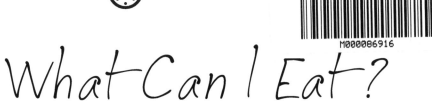

M000086916

What Can I Eat?
ON A
DAIRY FREE
DIET

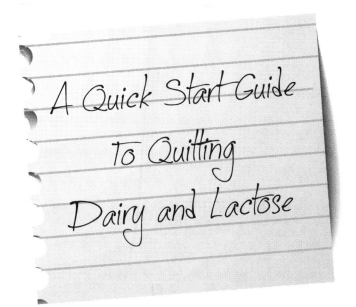

A Quick Start Guide To Quitting Dairy and Lactose

Lose Weight, Feel Great and Increase Your Energy!

PLUS 100 Delicious Dairy-Free Recipes

First published in 2015 by Erin Rose Publishing

Text and illustration copyright © 2015 Erin Rose Publishing

Design: Julie Anson

ISBN: 978-0-9928232-6-9

A CIP record for this book is available from the British Library.

DISCLAIMER: This book is for informational purposes only and not intended as a substitute for the medical advice, diagnosis or treatment of a physician or qualified healthcare provider. The reader should consult a physician before undertaking a new health care regimen and in all matters relating to his/her health, and particularly with respect to any symptoms that may require diagnosis or medical attention.

While every care has been taken in compiling the recipes for this book we cannot accept responsibility for any problems which arise as a result of preparing one of the recipes. The author and publisher disclaim responsibility for any adverse effects that may arise from the use or application of the recipes in this book. Some of the recipes in this book include nuts and eggs. If you have an egg or nut allergy it's important to avoid these. It is recommended that children, pregnant women, the elderly or anyone who has an immune system disorder avoid eating raw eggs.

CONTENTS

Recipes

Lunch

Dinner 63

Desserts, Sweet Treats & Snacks 99

Sauces & Condiments 113

INTRODUCTION

If you have just discovered that you are allergic or intolerant to lactose, a sugar found in goats, sheep and cow's milk then this **Quick Start Guide** is for you. Maybe you're relieved to find out that the cause of your unpleasant or embarrassing digestive problems, or that recurring skin complaint has been an allergy or intolerance to dairy produce and that it's avoidable. However, you may be thinking, 'Now what can I eat?' and feel daunted about how this will affect your diet and lifestyle. You aren't alone.

It's estimated that 75% of the world's population are affected by lactose intolerance which arises when we lack the ability to digest lactose, a sugar found in dairy products. It's common but its effects can be far reaching and in severe cases can cause life-threatening anaphylaxis. The concern for many people is that by removing dairy products from their diet they won't absorb enough calcium and they risk osteoporosis and weak bones. That needn't be the case. Recent research shows that beyond a certain amount of calcium which is easily attainable from other foods, no extra benefit was shown from consuming large quantities of dairy produce.

What's to Gain From Cutting Out Lactose?

Removing lactose from your diet or reducing your lactose intake could improve problems such as stomach cramps and bloating, recurrent skin rashes and nasal congestion, even in those who are only mildly affected by the lactose. People often find that cutting out or reducing lactose improves their skin condition or decreases mucous production and studies suggest reducing lactose consumption offers long term protection against certain types of cancers. And for the lactose intolerant, skipping dairy produce can provide relief from distressing and uncomfortable digestive symptoms and an improvement in their general wellbeing.

Basically, lactose intolerance occurs when we don't have the lactase enzyme required to digest the milk sugar, lactose. Many people lose the ability to digest lactose as they become adults and stress on the immune system also plays a role, as does a person's ethnicity. Lactose intolerance may not be reversible but it can be managed by changing your diet. However, that requires you having essential information to enable you to completely remove lactose from your diet. Some of us benefit from reducing our lactose intake, however if you're allergic and consuming it causes a severe reaction within minutes, you must avoid it entirely.

Apart from obvious sources of lactose like milk, yogurt and cream it's frequently found in many readymade foods and it's often an ingredient in prescription medication too, so it's wise to get informed.

The aim of this Quick Start Guide is to comprehensively provide you with the important information on why and how to go about removing dairy products and all lactose from your diet. Also in this book, we have included tips on how to make it easy, provided essential lists of what you can and can't eat, with insight into how to read the labels and find hidden lactose in pre-prepared food products. Plus, to really get you started, we've included 100 delicious and easy recipes which are easy to incorporate into a busy lifestyle. Our symptom checker provides you with a useful guide to how lactose could be affecting you, and if you're reading this book then the chances are you suspect that it is.

Often people have been on a frustrating quest, visiting professionals and seeking answers before they come to the conclusion that self-help is the only option. But don't worry, that puts you in control, and once you master the basics, being dairy-free will become natural for you.

Many people have found that after removing dairy from their diet their IBS, eczema, asthma, bloating and migraines vastly improve. Studies have also linked dairy consumption with increased risk of reproductive cancers, likely caused by IGF-1 which is growth factor found in cow's milk. The concentrations of IGF-1 have been found to be particularly high in prostate cancer, and women suffering from PCOS (Polycystic Ovaries Syndrome) often benefit from following a low dairy or dairy-free diet.

So for millions of people to achieve optimum health it makes sense to remove dairy from their diet. However, we don't want you to feel deprived or to miss out on your favourite dishes, so many of our recipes are for everyday meals which we've made dairy-free, taking into account that creamy dishes are not just tasty but the satisfying texture makes us feel like we've had something luxurious. So take control, and take action. You've taken the first step.

Skipping Dairy Products Causes Weak Bones - Fact or Fiction?

You can get all the calcium your body needs for healthy bones from sources other than dairy. You can also help prevent osteoporosis by taking simple steps such as reducing your sodium intake. Adequate calcium can be digested from green leafy vegetables and beans. It's proven that for adults and children, getting regular exercise increases bone density. Also make sure you are getting enough Vitamin D. Without it only 10% of calcium is absorbed. Vitamin D content in foods is low but other sources are sunlight and vitamin supplements.

Is Organic Milk Healthier?

Apart from synthetic bovine growth hormones which are given to cows to increase their milk production, milk also contains naturally occurring hormones from the cow; after all it is cow's breast milk. There are also concerns over the amount of antibiotics, which are used to treat mastitis, and pesticide toxins which are passed through the consumption of milk and can accumulate to harmful levels. However, one significant benefit or organic milk is that in organically farmed dairy cows the use of antibiotics is controlled.

Allergy Or Intolerance?

If you have already discovered that you're allergic to lactose it's imperative that you weed out all those sneaky lactose additions which creep into your everyday diet. Once you're in a pattern, you'll know the foods you can and can't have. However, if you suspect lactose is causing you health problems the first step is to consult your doctor, who can perform a test. Early diagnosis is essential for children to avoid repeated attacks of diarrhoea which can cause dehydration.

Even if your allergy test come back negative you could still have an intolerance to dairy and would benefit by removing it from your diet. There is an argument that a diet without dairy products, which contain calcium, protein and vitamins A and D, puts you at risk of malnutrition, however eating a wide variety of good, clean, healthy foods will ensure you gain what you need.

The lactose content of dairy foods differs depending on the fat content. Much of the lactose is lost in the liquid during processing. For instance butter, being largely fat, has much less lactose than milk. Therefore you may be alright to eat it if you have an intolerance, however not if you are allergic to lactose.

There are those who benefit from a reduction in dairy intake, whose symptoms may subside but return if their lactose consumption increases, therefore keeping a food diary can be incredibly helpful. The recipes in this book are dairy-free but please be vigilant when checking the ingredients on labels that lactose hasn't been unexpectedly added to some of your store cupboard basics.

Symptom Checker

Lactose affects us in different ways and this list isn't intended for medical diagnosis, but it is an indicator of the possible ways it could be affecting you. Consult your doctor first, but if your symptoms are unexplained it's worth removing lactose to see if there is an improvement

- Stomach pain and cramps
- Bloating
- Diarrhoea
- Constipation
- Vomiting
- Excessive gas
- Acne
- Chronic ear infections
- Sinus problems
- Hives
- Dry skin
- Eczema
- Psoriasis
- IBS
- Asthma
- Nasal congestion and excess mucous

If you have recurring digestive symptoms please consult your doctor who will check for underlying health conditions.

Can't I Just Take A Lactase Supplement?

It may seem obvious that if you aren't producing sufficient lactase enzymes, therefore having trouble digesting lactose, that taking a lactase supplement before eating dairy products will help you to digest it, however this isn't a cure. It depends how much lactose you are consuming as to how much lactase you need to supplement, and this can be incredibly difficult to gauge if you're eating out. It works for some but may not alleviate digestive symptoms completely. The lactase supplement has to be taken before eating your meal and many people find that socially awkward, it can require some planning and it doesn't eliminate the symptoms completely.

It can also be difficult to switch back and forward between being dairy-free and not being dairy-free, making it harder to avoid the foods which cause the symptoms.

Note that lactase supplements can trigger allergic reactions in some people, so if you experience tightness of your chest, difficulty breathing or urticaria (hives) get medical attention as soon as possible. For some people lactase supplements can work but many people simply prefer to avoid anything dairy and it's possible to obtain sufficient calcium from other foods without relying on dairy products.

Lactose free milk has been treated with the lactase enzyme to break it down, however if you are allergic to milk, as opposed to being intolerant, you should not consume lactose-free milk as it contains the proteins that cause allergies.

How Much Lactose Is Too Much?

Generally speaking, the closer a product is to milk the higher the lactose content will be, and the higher the fat content the lower will be the amount of lactose contained in it. If you are mildly lactose intolerant you may be able to have a small amount of it in your diet. Trace amounts of lactose may be tolerated depending on what your threshold is so try experimenting, unless of course you are severely allergic, in which case, avoid it. Butter does contain beneficial amounts of fat soluble vitamins including vitamins, A, E and K2.

Approximate Lactose Content Of Dairy Products

- Whey 39-78%
- Milk powder 36-52%
- Ice cream 6%
- Reduced fat milk 4-5%
- Full fat milk 4-5%
- Yogurt 4.5%
- Whipping cream 3%
- Mozzarella cheese 1-3%
- Cheddar cheese 0.07%
- Feta cheese 0-5%
- Butter 0.01%

What Can I Eat?

Don't Eat these:

All dairy products containing lactose, including:

- Milk

- Butter

- Yogurt

- Cream

- Cheese

- Whey

- Whey protein

- Ice cream

- Yogurt

- Buttermilk

- Fromage frais

- Ghee

- Skimmed milk powder

AVOID ALL PRODUCTS CONTAINING DAIRY AND/OR LACTOSE, CHECKING THE INGREDIENTS LIST

- Crème caramel

- Batter

- Cheesy crackers and biscuits

- Custard

- Artificial creams

Don't Eat these:

- Creamy desserts and puddings
- Bread
- Biscuits
- Cakes
- Pancakes
- Scones
- Pastries
- Chocolate
- Sweets
- Cheese flavoured crisps and snacks
- Readymade sauces such as cheese sauce, béchamel and other milk based sauces
- Low-fat spreads & margarine

What Can I Eat?

You Can Eat These:

- Soya milk

- Coconut milk

- Coconut cream

- Rice milk

- Almond milk

- Hazelnut milk

- Hemp milk

- Oat milk

- Soya yogurt

- Soya cheese

- Soya cream

- Dairy-free spreads

- Tahini (sesame seeds are very high in calcium)

- Chicken, lamb, beef, pork, fish and seafood

- Rice, quinoa, couscous, potatoes, pasta

- All fresh vegetables

- All fresh fruit

- Pulses, lentils, nuts and seeds

- Nut butters, such as peanut butter, almond butter and cashew nut butter

- Olive oil, ground nut oil

- Spices and fresh herbs

Don't Miss Out on Calcium

In the UK, the recommended daily intake of calcium for adults is 700mg, and 1000mg in the USA with the requirement for calcium increasing during adolescence and breast feeding. It's a common belief that we only obtain sufficient calcium from dairy products, however calcium is amply available in a wide range of foods. Apart from being a constituent of healthy bones, calcium is important for muscle contraction, nerve impulses and the secretion of hormones. Eating a varied diet with plenty of green leafy vegetables, such as kale, spinach, watercress, broccoli, pulses, whole grains, nuts, fruit and seeds will provide you with what you need. To help guide you we have included a list of the calcium contents of some foods to give you an idea what you need to get sufficient nutrients in your diet.

Vitamin D plays a valuable role in our ability to absorb calcium and getting plenty of sunlight is also important. It's recommended that around 20 minutes of sun a day on the face and arms is required to obtain sufficient vitamin D. This isn't easy to achieve in countries where sunshine is in limited supply and winters are so cold and dark. To ensure you get plenty of vitamin D eat plenty of eggs, liver and oily fish. Good quality supplements are also available. More and more research is discovering a link between vitamin D deficiency and chronic illnesses and it's thought that previous recommended requirements of the sunshine vitamin were not high enough.

Sources Of Calcium

Approximate Calcium Contents of Foods Per 100g

- Sesame seeds 975mg
- Sardines 382mg
- Almonds 264mg
- Brazil nuts 160mg
- Kale 150mg
- Parsley 138mg
- Black eyed peas 126mg
- Watercress 120mg
- Soya beans (cooked) 102mg
- Hazel nuts 114mg
- Pinto beans 113mg
- Wholemeal bread 107mg
- Chickpeas 105mg
- Spinach 99mg
- Okra 82mg
- Raisins 50mg
- Eggs 50mg
- Broccoli 47mg
- Brussels sprouts 42mg
- Oranges 40mg
- Dates 39mg
- Cashew nuts 37mg
- Lettuce 36mg
- Kidney beans 35mg
- Soya milk 25mg
- Onions 23mg
- Coconut milk 16mg
- Apricots 13mg

How To Read The Labels

Lactose can be found on food labels under the following names:

- Milk, milk powder, skimmed milk powder

- Butter, butterfat, butter solids, butter extract

- Dairy product solids, milk solids, milk sugar solids

- Whipping cream/sour cream

- Cheese and cheese powder

- Curds

- Low fat spreads and margarines

- Caramel

- Coffee whiteners/ creamers

- Malt drinks

- Condensed milk

- Quark

- Whey syrup, whey protein

- Casein, caseinates, sodium caseinate, hydrolysed casein, iron caseinate, zinc caseinate, calcium caseinate, ammonium caseinate

- Lactic acid (E270)

- Lactate solids

- Lactic yeast

- Lactalbumin, lactalbumin phosphate

- Lactulose

- Lactoglobulin

Top Tips To Make It Easy

Get Prepared, Get Started

- Clear your cupboards of products containing dairy, making sure you check all the labels.

- Stock up with dairy-free snacks. Avocados, nuts, seeds and olives are quick and easy snacks which are handy to keep you going until the next meal.

- Experiment with different dairy-free milks until you find your favourite. Rice milk is fairly sweet and goes well in cereals and drinks whereas soya milk is better in savoury dishes as it's creamy.

- Go cold turkey! Eliminating dairy produce, even for a short while gives you a chance to monitor your changes.

- Keep a food diary. It will not only help you keep track of what you are eating, but also record your how you feel which will give you an insight into any patterns which may exist.

- Experiment with the recipes and find your favourites.

- Plan meals that you can look forward to so you won't feel deprived. Eliminating dairy isn't a punishment. It's a way of eating that rewards you with good health.

- Check your medication for lactose and ask your pharmacist if you're not sure.

- Cosmetics, soaps, lotions and creams may also contain milk. This may not be a problem for many but for the highly allergic it can be.

- Check your vitamin and mineral supplements don't contain lactose.

- Prepare some tasty meals and treats for the fridge or freezer. Have something dairy-free close by so that you aren't tempted. Carrying a packet of nuts not only curbs hunger cravings but they will boost of nutrients, especially calcium.

Cheat Sheet

Going dairy-free gives you the chance to be more creative with your meals and below are some tasty alternatives to your usual dairy options.

- Chopped or grated (shredded) Brazil nuts or sunflower seeds ground in a blender make a tasty alternative to a cheesy topping and can be used instead of cheese on salads, soups or pie toppings.

- Coconut cream as a substitute for whipped cream.

- Add a smooth nut butter like cashew nut butter or peanut butter into sauces and curries for creamy nutty flavours.

- Spread hummus or guacamole onto sandwiches and wraps instead of butter or cheese. Thankfully home-made guacamole is simple to make as shop bought guacamole can have cream added.

- Add slices of avocado to salads for the rich creamy texture of cheese.

- Oatmeal can even be made with water and rice or almond milk added later.

- Courgette (zucchini) or potato added to soups, stews or casseroles can make it richer and creamier tasting.

- Try adding soya milk to savoury dishes which require a creamy texture

- For sweet dishes, drinks and pour-overs for cereals, almond milk and rice milk taste sweeter although rice milk has a more watery consistency.

- A combination of two different dairy-free milks can work really well, especially for a sugar-free hot chocolate. Combine soya milk and rice milk in equal quantities before adding a small teaspoon of 100% cocoa powder. The rice milk reduces the need for extra sweetness.

- If a recipe requires milk powder you can use rice flour, potato flour, soya or coconut flour instead.

Recipes

Simple Recipes That Make Going Dairy-Free Easy!

The recipes in this book are easy to fit into a busy schedule, simple to follow and very tasty. We don't want you to feel deprived when you give up lactose. On the contrary, by reducing your lactose intake it'll open you up to other interesting food possibilities that your taste buds will really enjoy.

Experimenting is the key, and finding out what works for you. Once your kitchen cupboards are stocked with what you like, you can play around with the recipes and find your favourites. Get creative and make it easier for yourself, put the right kind of temptation in your way: include in your diet something which you can really look forward too. Coconut milk is an amazing alternative to dairy milk and is a great store cupboard staple to add to so many great dishes.

Dairy-free milk alternatives like soya milk, rice milk, almond milk etc. have a long shelf life so once you have discovered what works best for you, you'll be able to stock up. The best way to know that what you are eating is lactose free is to make your own food from scratch. It may not take as much time as you think. By using fresh whole foods, you won't need to worry about what's been added to ready-made meals. To begin with you'll be re-training your taste buds but it won't be long until being dairy-free is easy.

We wish you good luck, good health and we hope you enjoy the recipes!

BREAKFAST

Spiced Scrambled Egg

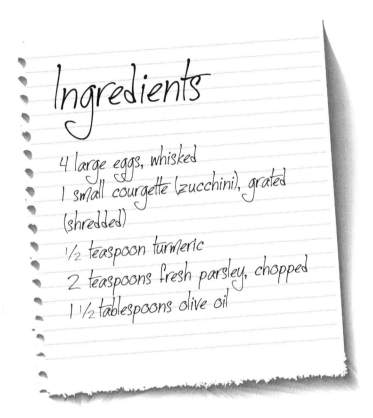

Ingredients

4 large eggs, whisked
1 small courgette (zucchini), grated (shredded)
½ teaspoon turmeric
2 teaspoons fresh parsley, chopped
1½ tablespoons olive oil

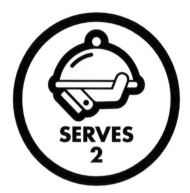

SERVES
2

Method

Heat the oil in a frying pan, sprinkle in the turmeric and stir. Add the courgette (zucchini) to the pan and cook for 2 minutes. Pour in the beaten eggs and stir the mixture until it's lightly scrambled. Sprinkle with parsley and serve.

Leek & Spinach Frittata

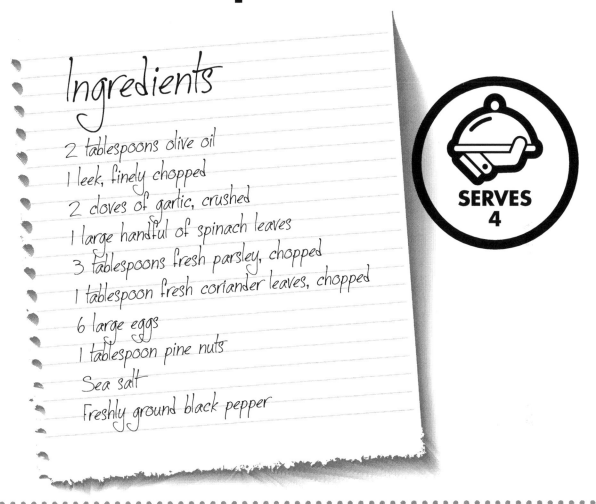

Ingredients

2 tablespoons olive oil

1 leek, finely chopped

2 cloves of garlic, crushed

1 large handful of spinach leaves

3 tablespoons fresh parsley, chopped

1 tablespoon fresh coriander leaves, chopped

6 large eggs

1 tablespoon pine nuts

Sea salt

Freshly ground black pepper

SERVES 4

Method

Heat half of the olive oil in a frying pan and add the garlic and leeks. Cook for around 5 minutes, until soft. Whisk the eggs in a large bowl. Add the leeks, garlic, spinach, pine nuts and herbs. Season with salt and pepper. Heat the remaining olive oil in a pan. Pour in the egg mixture and cook until the eggs becomes firm. Place the frying pan under a hot grill for 2 minutes to make sure the top of the frittata is cooked. Can be served warm or cold so this can be made in advance and eaten for breakfast or lunch on the go.

Baked Eggs & Smoked Salmon

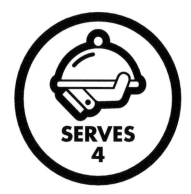

SERVES 4

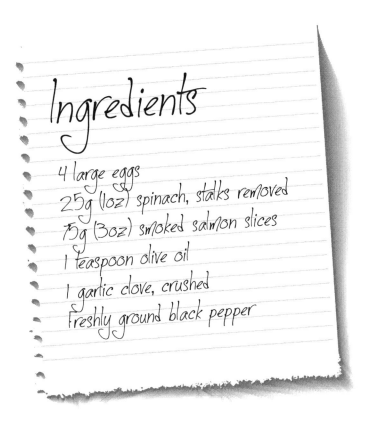

Ingredients

4 large eggs
25g (1oz) spinach, stalks removed
75g (3oz) smoked salmon slices
1 teaspoon olive oil
1 garlic clove, crushed
Freshly ground black pepper

Method

Heat the olive oil in a pan and add the garlic. When the garlic starts to soften, add the spinach. Cook for 2-3 minutes until the spinach has wilted. Line the bases and sides of 4 ramekin dishes with smoked salmon. Divide the spinach and the garlic between the ramekin dishes then break an egg into each one. Sprinkle with black pepper. Place the ramekins in a preheated oven at 220C/425F for 15 minutes, until the eggs are set. Serve and enjoy.

Granola

Ingredients

- 225g (8oz) oats
- 60g (2½ oz) Brazil nuts, chopped
- 60g (2½ oz) almond flakes
- 60g (2½ oz) sunflower seeds
- 2 tablespoons honey
- 2 tablespoons coconut oil or olive oil
- 3 tablespoons water
- 1 teaspoon cinnamon
- ½ teaspoon ginger
- 125g (4oz) mixed dried fruit; raisins, apricots, cranberries or dates

Method

Place the oats, sunflower seeds, almond flakes and nuts into a bowl and mix well. In a separate bowl stir together the oil, honey, cinnamon, ginger and water. Add the oats, seeds and nuts and combine. Scatter the mixture onto a baking tray and bake in the oven at 190C/375F for 30 minutes, until crisp and golden. Remove and allow it to cool. Mix in the dried fruit and store in a container until ready to use. Serve with non-dairy milk, such as almond, soya, oat or rice milk.

Chicken & Tomato Omelette

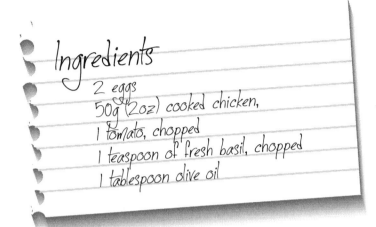

Ingredients

2 eggs
50g (2oz) cooked chicken,
1 tomato, chopped
1 teaspoon of fresh basil, chopped
1 tablespoon olive oil

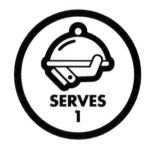

SERVES
1

Method

Put the eggs in a small bowl and whisk. Stir in the basil, chicken and tomato. Warm the oil in a small frying pan and add the beaten egg mixture. Cook for 1 minute and allow it to start to set without stirring. Continue cooking until the eggs are set firm.

Pear Porridge

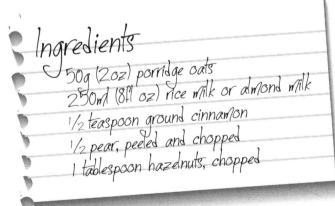

Ingredients

50g (2oz) porridge oats
250ml (8fl oz) rice milk or almond milk
1/2 teaspoon ground cinnamon
1/2 pear, peeled and chopped
1 tablespoon hazelnuts, chopped

SERVES
1

Method

In a saucepan, cook all the ingredients, apart from nuts, for 5 minutes or until it thickens. Serve topped with nuts and a little honey if required.

Spinach & Apple Smoothie

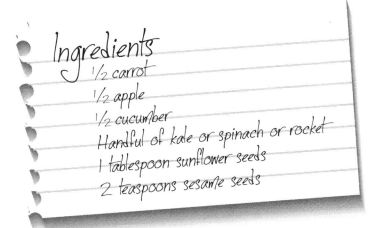

Ingredients
- ½ carrot
- ½ apple
- ½ cucumber
- Handful of kale or spinach or rocket
- 1 tablespoon sunflower seeds
- 2 teaspoons sesame seeds

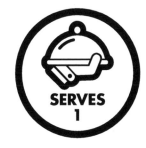

SERVES 1

Method

Place all the ingredients into a blender and around a cup of water. Blitz until smooth. You can add a little extra water if you don't want it too thick.

Raspberry & Coconut Smoothie

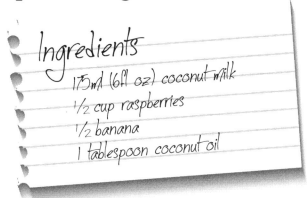

Ingredients
- 175ml (6fl oz) coconut milk
- ½ cup raspberries
- ½ banana
- 1 tablespoon coconut oil

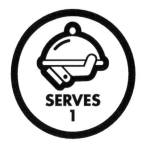

SERVES 1

Method

Toss all of the ingredients into a blender. Blitz until creamy. Pour and enjoy!

Pineapple & Cucumber Smoothie

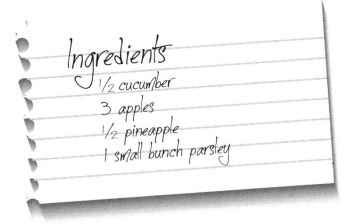

Ingredients
- ½ cucumber
- 3 apples
- ½ pineapple
- 1 small bunch parsley

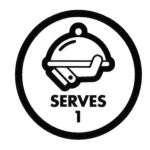

SERVES
1

Method

Place all the ingredients into a smoothie maker or blender and blitz until smooth.

Avocado & Orange Smoothie

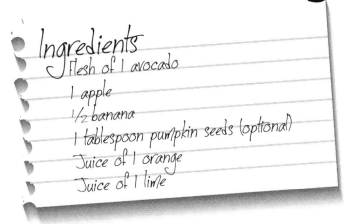

Ingredients
- Flesh of 1 avocado
- 1 apple
- ½ banana
- 1 tablespoon pumpkin seeds (optional)
- Juice of 1 orange
- Juice of 1 lime

SERVES
1

Method

Put all the ingredients into a blender with just enough water to cover the ingredients. Blitz until smooth. It's frothy and delicious.

Warm Raspberry Soufflé Omelette

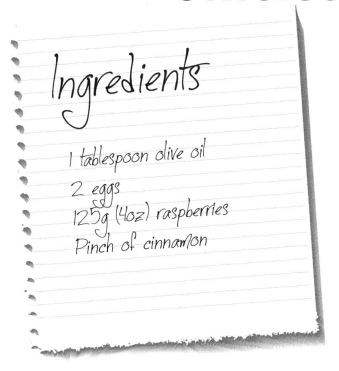

Ingredients

1 tablespoon olive oil

2 eggs

125g (4oz) raspberries

Pinch of cinnamon

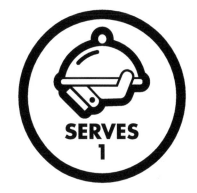

**SERVES
1**

Method

Heat the fruit in a saucepan for 5 minutes and mash with a fork. Stir in a sprinkling of cinnamon. Set aside. Separate the egg yolks from the whites. Keep the yolks in a separate bowl while you whisk the egg whites into peaks. Then fold the yolks into the egg whites.

Heat the oil in a small frying pan and add the eggs. Cook the omelette until the eggs have set. It should be light and fluffy. Serve open on a plate, add the raspberries and fold over. Eat straight away.

Pancakes

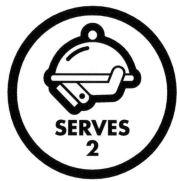

**SERVES
2**

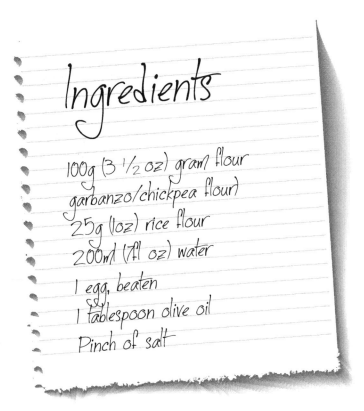

Ingredients

100g (3 ½ oz) gram flour
garbanzo/chickpea flour)
25g (1oz) rice flour
200ml (7fl oz) water
1 egg, beaten
1 tablespoon olive oil
Pinch of salt

Method

Place the gram flour and rice flour, salt, egg and water into a blender and process until smooth. Or alternatively combine the ingredients in a bowl. Allow the mixture to stand for 10 minutes. Heat the olive oil in a frying pan. Add a little of the pancake mixture into the pan and cook for 2 or 3 minutes on each side. The mixture should make 4 large pancakes or 8 small ones.

Note: This recipe uses gluten-free flour but you can substitute it for plain flour.

Herby Courgette (Zucchini) Frittata

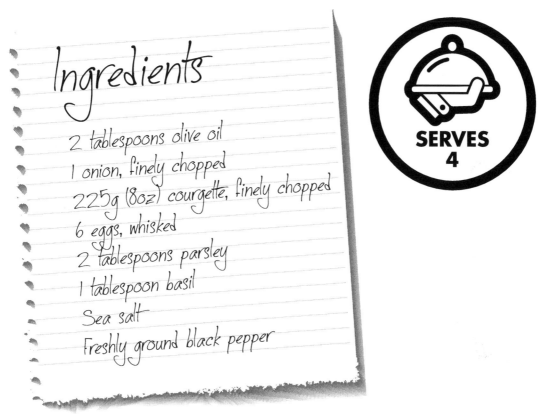

Ingredients

2 tablespoons olive oil

1 onion, finely chopped

225g (8oz) courgette, finely chopped

6 eggs, whisked

2 tablespoons parsley

1 tablespoon basil

Sea salt

Freshly ground black pepper

SERVES 4

Method

Heat the olive oil in a frying pan. Add the onion and cook for 4-5 minutes to soften. Add the courgette (zucchini) and cook for 3-4 minutes. Pour the beaten eggs into the pan and season with salt and pepper. Sprinkle with the herbs. Cook for 3 minutes until set and cooked around the edge. Finish off under the grill for 1-2 minutes until cooked thoroughly. Serve and enjoy.

LUNCH

Quick Curried Prawns

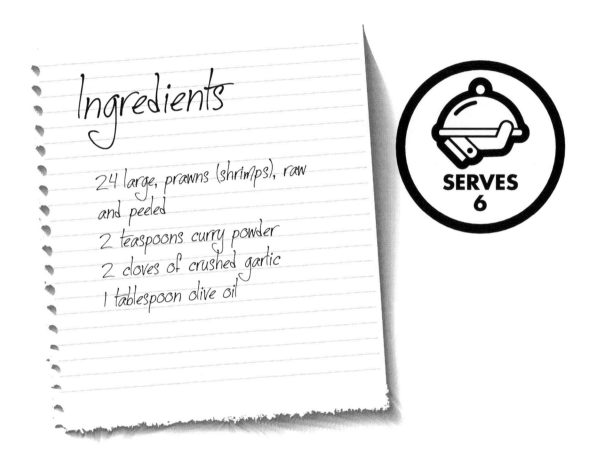

Ingredients

24 large, prawns (shrimps), raw and peeled
2 teaspoons curry powder
2 cloves of crushed garlic
1 tablespoon olive oil

SERVES 6

Method

Heat the oil in a frying pan. Add the curry powder and garlic then stir. Add the prawns. Cook for 3 to 5 minutes on each side, or until the prawns are completely pink and cooked thoroughly. Transfer them to a serving dish and pour the oil over them. Serve with rice and salad.

Roasted Red Pepper Soup (Bell Pepper)

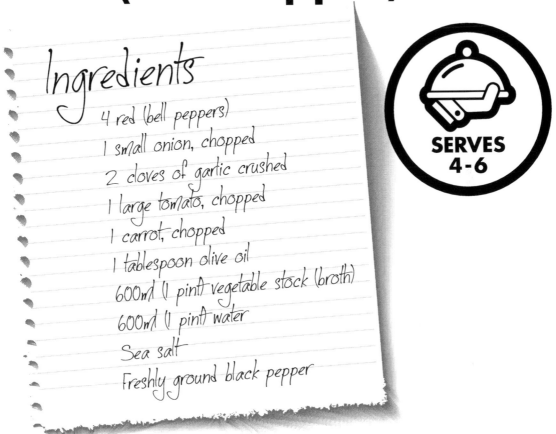

Ingredients

- 4 red (bell peppers)
- 1 small onion, chopped
- 2 cloves of garlic crushed
- 1 large tomato, chopped
- 1 carrot, chopped
- 1 tablespoon olive oil
- 600ml (1 pint) vegetable stock (broth)
- 600ml (1 pint) water
- Sea salt
- Freshly ground black pepper

SERVES 4-6

Method

Heat a grill (broiler) and place the peppers underneath. Keep turning them until they are browned on all side. Remove them from the heat and carefully remove the skins, seeds and stalks then set aside. Heat the oil in a saucepan and add the onion and garlic. Cook for 4 minutes. Add in the tomatoes, carrot, red peppers, water and stock (broth). Bring to the boil, reduce the heat and simmer for 30 minutes. Use a hand blender or food processor and blitz the soup until smooth. Season with salt and pepper. Serve and enjoy.

Cream of Mushroom Soup

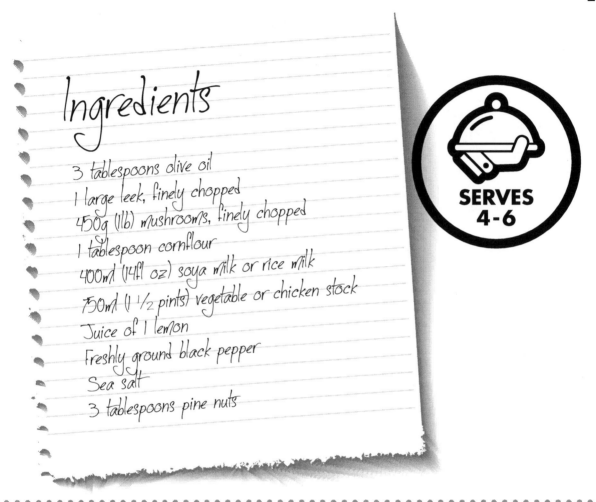

Ingredients

3 tablespoons olive oil
1 large leek, finely chopped
450g (1lb) mushrooms, finely chopped
1 tablespoon cornflour
400ml (14fl oz) soya milk or rice milk
750ml (1 ½ pints) vegetable or chicken stock
Juice of 1 lemon
Freshly ground black pepper
Sea salt
3 tablespoons pine nuts

SERVES 4-6

Method

Heat the olive oil in a saucepan. Add the leeks and mushrooms and cook for 15 minutes or until the vegetables are soft. Sprinkle in the cornflour and stir. Pour in the soya or rice milk together with the stock. Bring to the boil, cover and simmer gently for 30 minutes. Blend the soup until smooth. Return to the heat if necessary. Stir in the lemon juice and season with salt and pepper. In a frying pan, dry toast the pine nuts until they are slightly golden. Sprinkle onto the soup just before serving.

Butternut Squash & Ginger Soup

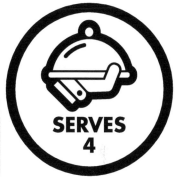

SERVES 4

Ingredients

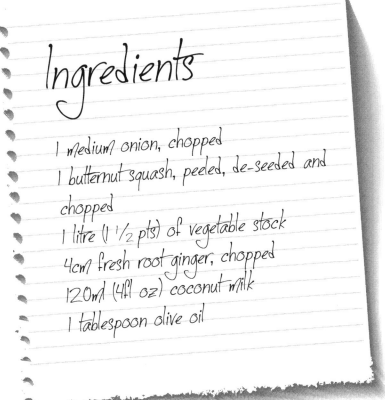

1 medium onion, chopped

1 butternut squash, peeled, de-seeded and chopped

1 litre (1 ½ pts) of vegetable stock

4cm fresh root ginger, chopped

120ml (4fl oz) coconut milk

1 tablespoon olive oil

Method

In a large saucepan, heat the olive oil and add the onion. Cook for 4 minutes, until the onion begins to soften. Add the squash, ginger and vegetable stock and bring to the boil. Reduce the heat and cook for 15 minutes, until the squash is soft. Pour the soup into a blender and blitz until smooth. Stir in the coconut milk. Return to the heat and warm through then serve.

Cauliflower Soup

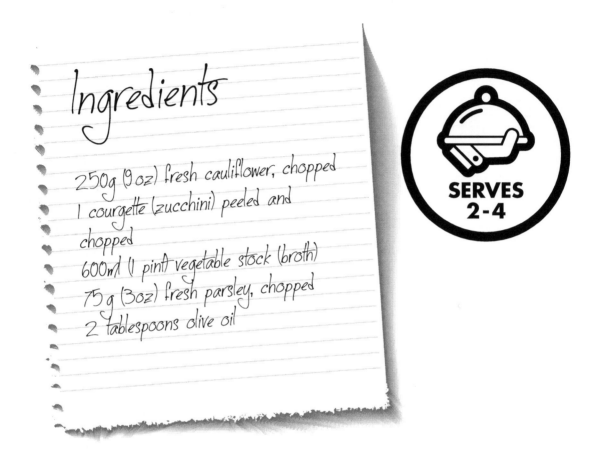

Ingredients

250g (9 oz) fresh cauliflower, chopped
1 courgette (zucchini) peeled and chopped
600ml (1 pint) vegetable stock (broth)
75g (3oz) fresh parsley, chopped
2 tablespoons olive oil

SERVES 2-4

Method

Heat the olive oil in a large saucepan and add the cauliflower and courgette (zucchini). Cook for around 5 minutes, stirring occasionally. Add the stock (broth), and simmer gently for 15 minutes. Pour the soup into a blender, add the parsley and blitz until smooth. Return the soup to the saucepan and gently simmer for 5 minutes to heat it through.

Leek & Potato Soup

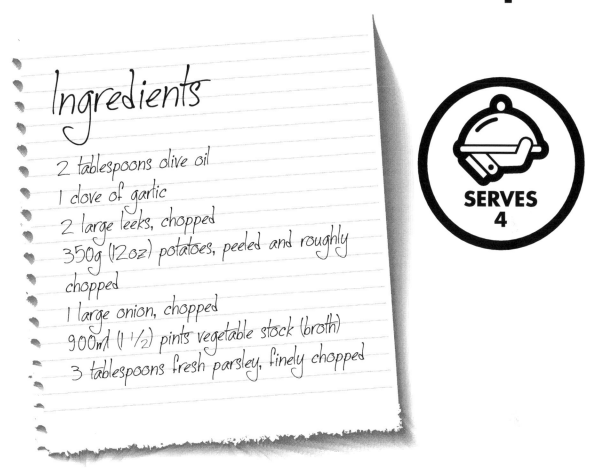

Ingredients

2 tablespoons olive oil
1 clove of garlic
2 large leeks, chopped
350g (12oz) potatoes, peeled and roughly chopped
1 large onion, chopped
900ml (1 1/2) pints vegetable stock (broth)
3 tablespoons fresh parsley, finely chopped

SERVES 4

Method

Heat the oil in a large saucepan. Add the garlic, potatoes, leeks and onions. Stir and cook for 10 minutes. Add in the vegetable stock (broth) and simmer for 25 minutes. Use a hand blender or food processor and liquidise the soup. Season and sprinkle with parsley before serving.

Chicken Soup

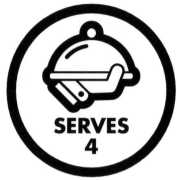

SERVES
4

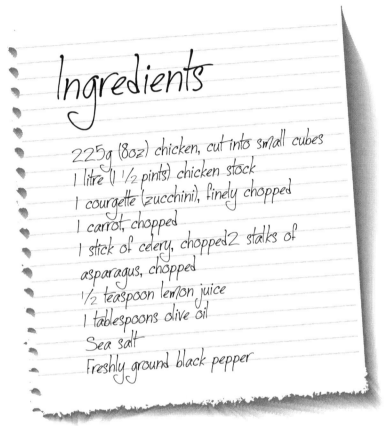

Ingredients

225g (8oz) chicken, cut into small cubes
1 litre (1 1/2 pints) chicken stock
1 courgette (zucchini), finely chopped
1 carrot, chopped
1 stick of celery, chopped 2 stalks of
asparagus, chopped
1/2 teaspoon lemon juice
1 tablespoons olive oil
Sea salt
Freshly ground black pepper

Method

Heat the olive oil in a frying pan. Add the chicken and cook for 10 minutes. Place the chicken, stock and lemon juice into a large saucepan. Cook for 5 minutes. Add the courgette (zucchini), carrot, celery and asparagus. Continue cooking for around 20 minutes, until the vegetables are soft. Season the soup with salt and pepper. Serve and eat immediately

Beetroot Soup

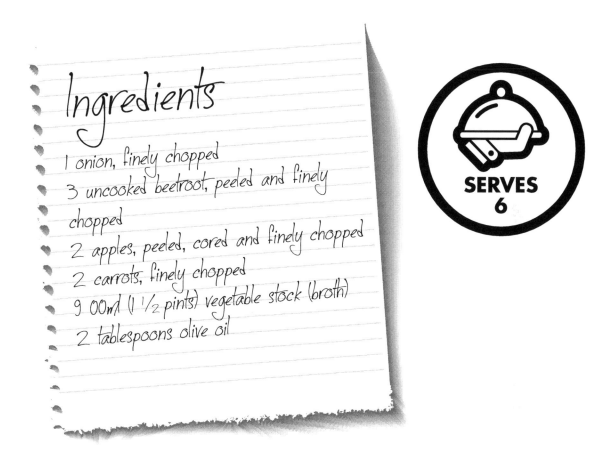

Ingredients

1 onion, finely chopped
3 uncooked beetroot, peeled and finely chopped
2 apples, peeled, cored and finely chopped
2 carrots, finely chopped
900ml (1 ½ pints) vegetable stock (broth)
2 tablespoons olive oil

SERVES 6

Method

Place the oil in a saucepan and add the onion. Cook for 5 minutes until it softens. Add in the beetroot and carrots to the saucepan and cook for 15 minutes. Add in the stock (broth) and apples. Bring to the boil, reduce the heat and simmer for 20 minutes. Blend the soup until smooth or serve as it is. Pour into bowls and enjoy.

Tomato & Basil Soup

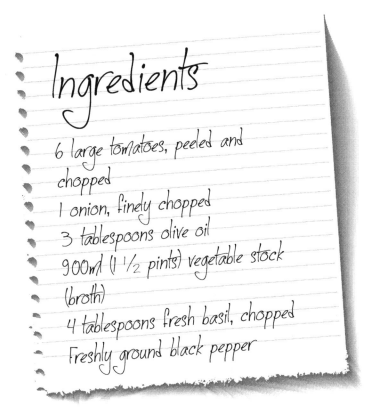

Ingredients

6 large tomatoes, peeled and chopped

1 onion, finely chopped

3 tablespoons olive oil

900ml (1 ½ pints) vegetable stock (broth)

4 tablespoons fresh basil, chopped

Freshly ground black pepper

SERVES 4

Method

Heat the oil in a saucepan and add the onion. Cook for 5 minutes until the onion softens. Add in the tomatoes and simmer gently until the tomatoes are soft and pulpy. Add the stock (broth) and cook for 5 minutes. Season with pepper and add 3 tablespoons of fresh basil. Blend in a liquidiser or use a hand blender and process until smooth. Stir in the remaining basil just before serving.

Sweet Potato & Tomato Soup

SERVES 4-6

Ingredients

1 large onion, chopped
300g (11oz) sweet potato, peeled and chopped
1 x 400g (14oz) tin chopped tomatoes
600ml 1 pint vegetable stock
1 tablespoon fresh coriander, chopped
1 tablespoon fresh parsley, chopped
1 tablespoon olive oil
Freshly ground black pepper
Sea salt

Method

Heat the olive oil in a saucepan and add the onions and sweet potatoes. Stir and cook for 5 minutes until the onion begins to soften. Add the stock (broth) and tomatoes. Bring to the boil, reduce the heat and simmer for 20 minutes. Stir in the herbs. Using a hand blender or food processor, blend until smooth. If the soup seems too thick, thin it down with a little extra stock or hot water. Season with salt and pepper. Serve and enjoy.

Thai Chicken Noodle Soup

Ingredients

150g (5oz) cooked chicken, shredded (leftovers are fine)
125g (4 oz) rice noodles,
100ml (3 ½ fl oz) coconut milk
1 tablespoon curry paste
2 onions
2 cloves of garlic, chopped
2 litres (3 pints) chicken stock (broth)
3 tablespoons fresh coriander (cilantro), chopped
Zest of 1 lime
1 tablespoon olive oil

SERVES 4-6

Method

Heat the oil in a saucepan. Add the curry paste and stir. Add in the garlic, onions and lime with a tablespoon of stock (broth). Cook for around 5 minutes until the onion has softened. Add to the saucepan the chicken, and the remaining stock. Bring to the boil then add the rice noodles. Reduce the heat and simmer for around 3 minutes or until the noodles are cooked. Stir in the coriander (cilantro) and coconut milk and warm it through. Season and serve.

Quick Chicken Casserole

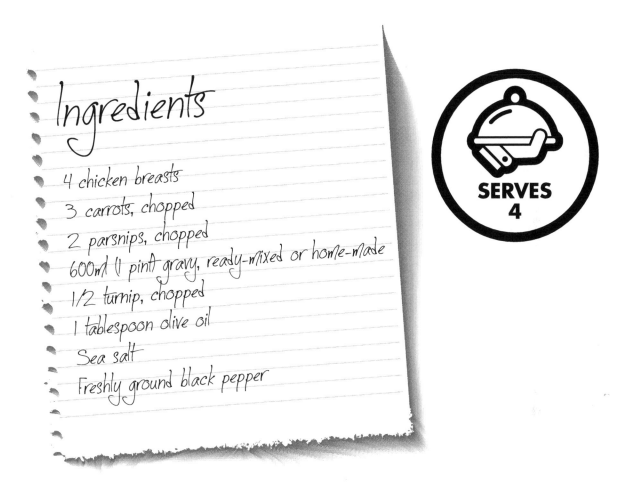

Ingredients

- 4 chicken breasts
- 3 carrots, chopped
- 2 parsnips, chopped
- 600ml (1 pint) gravy, ready-mixed or home-made
- 1/2 turnip, chopped
- 1 tablespoon olive oil
- Sea salt
- Freshly ground black pepper

SERVES 4

Method

Heat the oil in a large saucepan dish. Add the chicken and cook for 5 minutes. Add in the carrots, parsnip and turnip. Cook for around 15 minutes or until the vegetables are cooked. Add in the gravy and cook for 10 minutes. Season with salt and pepper before serving.

Thai Chicken Burgers

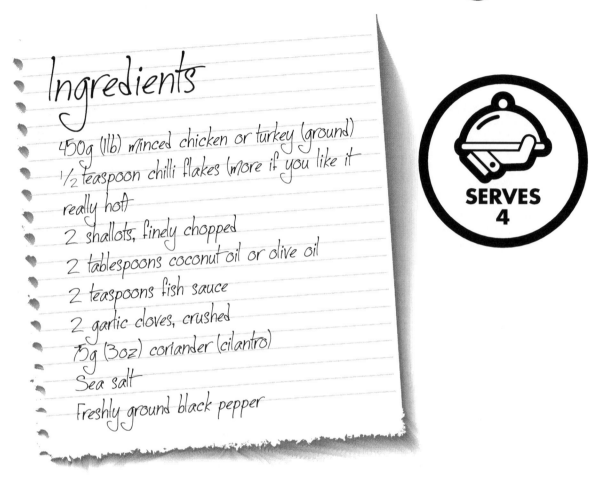

Ingredients

- 450g (1lb) minced chicken or turkey (ground)
- 1/2 teaspoon chilli flakes (more if you like it really hot)
- 2 shallots, finely chopped
- 2 tablespoons coconut oil or olive oil
- 2 teaspoons fish sauce
- 2 garlic cloves, crushed
- 75g (3oz) coriander (cilantro)
- Sea salt
- Freshly ground black pepper

SERVES 4

Method

Place the chicken in a large bowl and add the coriander (cilantro), fish sauce, garlic, shallots and chilli flakes. Season with salt and pepper. Mix the ingredients together well. Divide the mixture into 4 and form into burger shapes. Heat the oil in a frying pan. Place the burgers into the frying pan and cook for 7- 8 minutes on either side or until the burgers are cooked thoroughly.

Chicken Satay Skewers

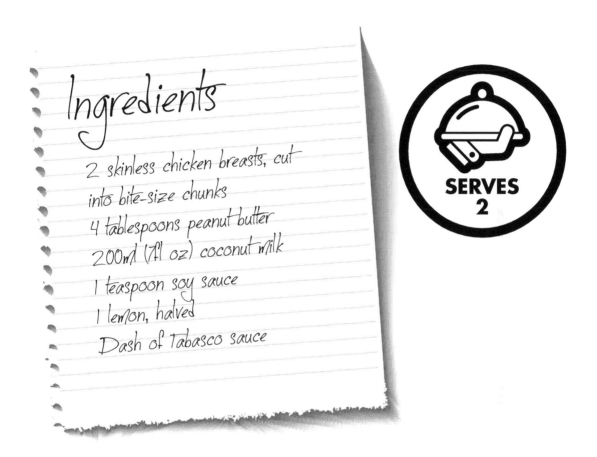

Ingredients

2 skinless chicken breasts, cut
into bite-size chunks
4 tablespoons peanut butter
200ml (7fl oz) coconut milk
1 teaspoon soy sauce
1 lemon, halved
Dash of Tabasco sauce

SERVES 2

Method

Put the peanut butter and coconut milk into a bowl and mix well. Add the Tabasco, soy sauce and stir. Place the chicken chunks into a bowl and pour the coconut and peanut sauce over it. Coat the chicken completely. Thread the chicken onto skewers, and set aside the remaining satay sauce. Place the chicken skewers under a hot grill (broiler) and cook for 4-5 minutes on each side or until cooked through. Place the remaining satay sauce in a small pan and add the juice from half a lemon. Bring the sauce to the boil. Cut the remaining lemon into 2 wedges. Serve the chicken skewers and pour the remaining satay sauce on top.

Chorizo & Tomato Hash

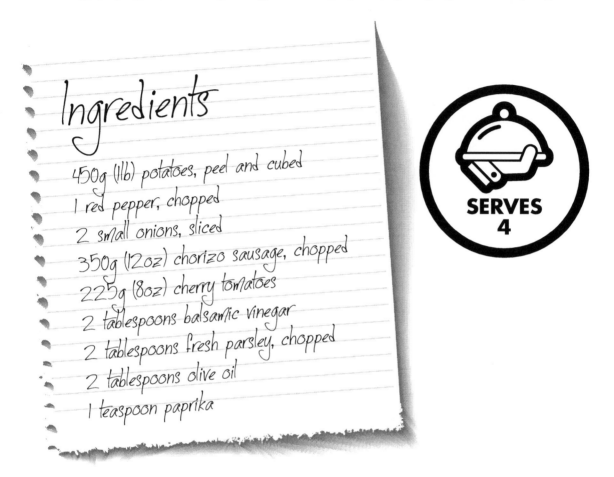

Ingredients

450g (1lb) potatoes, peel and cubed
1 red pepper, chopped
2 small onions, sliced
350g (12oz) chorizo sausage, chopped
225g (8oz) cherry tomatoes
2 tablespoons balsamic vinegar
2 tablespoons fresh parsley, chopped
2 tablespoons olive oil
1 teaspoon paprika

SERVES 4

Method

Heat the oil in a frying pan. Add the potatoes and cook until soft and slightly golden. Add in the red pepper (bell pepper) and onion. Cook for 5 minutes until softened. Sprinkle in the paprika and stir. Add in the chorizo, tomatoes and balsamic vinegar. Warm it thoroughly. Sprinkle with parsley and serve.

Burrito Lettuce Wrap

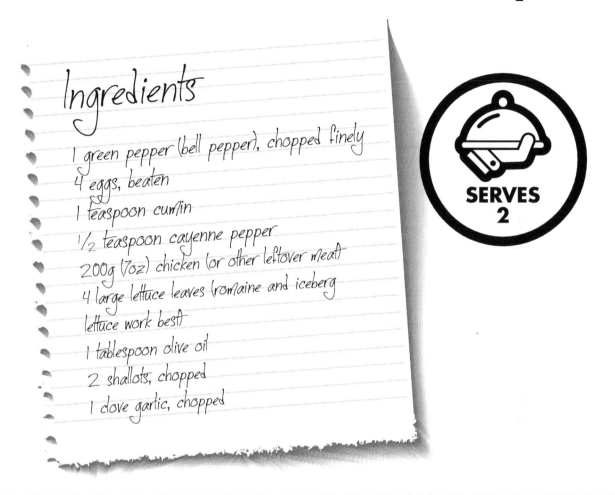

Ingredients

1 green pepper (bell pepper), chopped finely

4 eggs, beaten

1 teaspoon cumin

1/2 teaspoon cayenne pepper

200g (7oz) chicken (or other leftover meat)

4 large lettuce leaves (romaine and iceberg lettuce work best)

1 tablespoon olive oil

2 shallots, chopped

1 clove garlic, chopped

SERVES 2

Method

Heat the oil in a frying pan, add the shallots and garlic. Cook for 5 minutes, until soft. Add the green pepper, cumin, cayenne pepper and chicken and cook for around 3 minutes. Add the eggs and scramble everything together. Serve the filling wrapped in large lettuce leaves. It makes a low carb meal or you can of course serve in the traditional flour tortillas.

Creamy Pumpkin & Peanut Curry

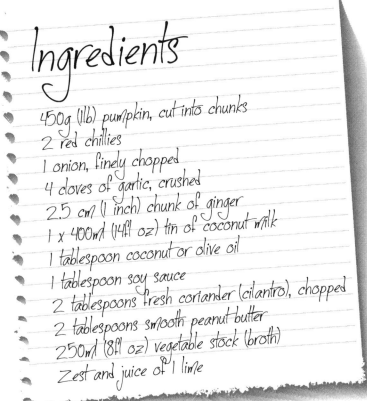

Ingredients

- 450g (1lb) pumpkin, cut into chunks
- 2 red chillies
- 1 onion, finely chopped
- 4 cloves of garlic, crushed
- 2.5 cm (1 inch) chunk of ginger
- 1 x 400ml (14fl oz) tin of coconut milk
- 1 tablespoon coconut or olive oil
- 1 tablespoon soy sauce
- 2 tablespoons fresh coriander (cilantro), chopped
- 2 tablespoons smooth peanut butter
- 250ml (8fl oz) vegetable stock (broth)
- Zest and juice of 1 lime

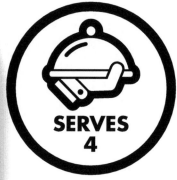

SERVES 4

Method

Heat the oil in a saucepan and add the onions and garlic. Cook for 5 minutes until the onion softens. Add in the ginger and chopped chillies. Stir well. Add the pumpkin, coriander (cilantro), soy sauce, peanut butter, lime zest and juice. Pour in the stock (broth). Bring to the boil, reduce the heat and simmer for 12-14 minutes, until the pumpkin has softened. Stir in the coconut milk and heat thoroughly. Season with salt and pepper. Serve with rice.

Fennel Salad

Ingredients

1 large fennel bulb, finely chopped

2 chicory bulbs, sliced

2 small lambs lettuce, chopped

3 spring onions (scallions) chopped

Zest of 1 large orange and the flesh chopped

3 tablespoons red wine vinegar

4 tablespoons olive oil

Sea salt

Freshly ground black pepper

SERVES 4

Method

Place the lettuce, chicory and spring onion (scallion) into a bowl. In a separate bowl mix together the olive oil, vinegar and orange zest. Mix the dressing well and season with salt and pepper. Place the fennel and orange flesh into the dressing and mix well. Pour the dressing, fennel and orange over the salad and toss it. Chill before serving.

Avocado & Pinto Bean Salad

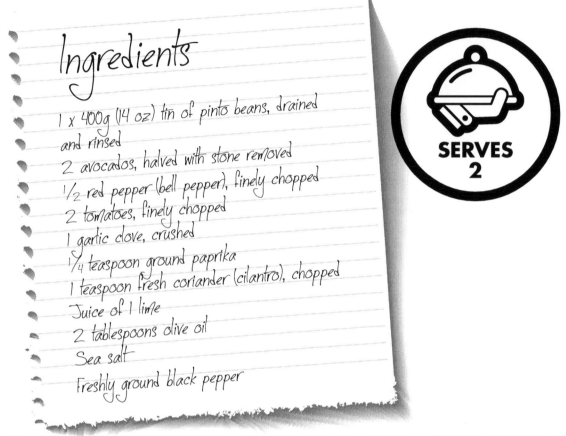

Ingredients

1 x 400g (14 oz) tin of pinto beans, drained and rinsed

2 avocados, halved with stone removed

1/2 red pepper (bell pepper), finely chopped

2 tomatoes, finely chopped

1 garlic clove, crushed

1/4 teaspoon ground paprika

1 teaspoon fresh coriander (cilantro), chopped

Juice of 1 lime

2 tablespoons olive oil

Sea salt

Freshly ground black pepper

SERVES 2

Method

To make the dressing, put the lime juice in a large bowl and whisk in the olive oil. Stir in the pinto beans, red pepper, tomatoes, coriander (cilantro), garlic, paprika, salt and black pepper. Mix together until everything is coated with the dressing. Place the avocado halves onto 4 plates and spoon the mixture over them. Serve and enjoy.

Chilli & Lime Turkey Strips

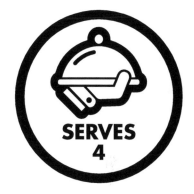

SERVES 4

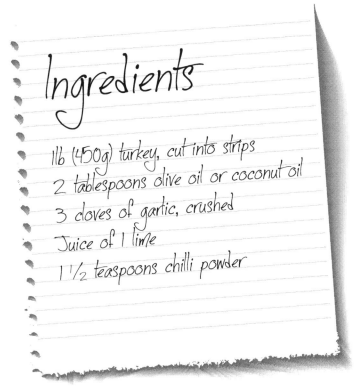

Ingredients

1lb (450g) turkey, cut into strips

2 tablespoons olive oil or coconut oil

3 cloves of garlic, crushed

Juice of 1 lime

1½ teaspoons chilli powder

Method

Heat the oil in a frying pan and add the turkey. Stir-fry the turkey for 2-3 minutes, then add the chilli powder, garlic and lime juice. Continue stirring for another 6 or 7 minutes or until cooked thoroughly. These are a versatile and tasty addition to rice, salads, stir fries and wraps.

Tuna & Bean Salad

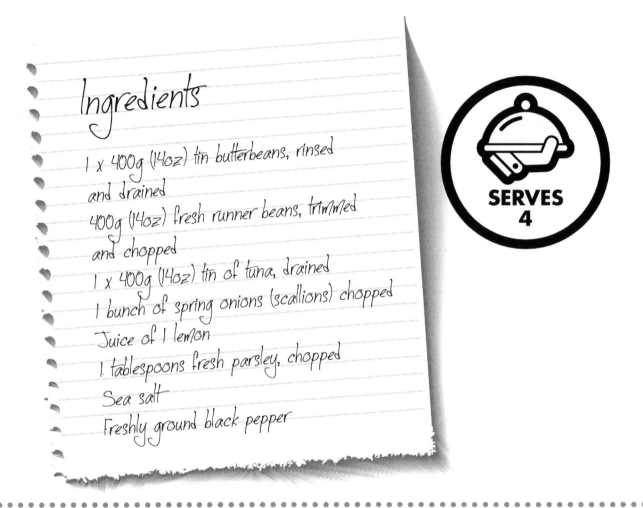

Ingredients

1 x 400g (14oz) tin butterbeans, rinsed and drained

400g (14oz) fresh runner beans, trimmed and chopped

1 x 400g (14oz) tin of tuna, drained

1 bunch of spring onions (scallions) chopped

Juice of 1 lemon

1 tablespoons fresh parsley, chopped

Sea salt

Freshly ground black pepper

SERVES 4

Method

Steam the runner beans for 5 minutes until they begin to soften. When the runner beans are cooked, place them in a bowl with the butterbeans and add the spring onions (scallions). Add to the bowl the tuna and mix it well. Squeeze in the lemon juice and season with salt and pepper. Serve with a sprinkling of fresh parsley.

Lemony Herb Quinoa Salad

Ingredients

250g (9 oz) quinoa, cooked
4 spring onions, (scallions), finely chopped
1/2 cucumber, peeled and diced
6 cherry tomatoes, quartered
2 tablespoons fresh basil, finely chopped
2 tablespoons fresh coriander, (cilantro), finely chopped
2 tablespoons fresh parsley, finely chopped
6 pitted olives, finely chopped
60ml (2fl oz) olive oil
2 cloves garlic, crushed
Juice of 2 lemons
Sea salt
Freshly ground black pepper

SERVES 2

Method

In a large bowl, mix together the garlic, olive oil, lemon juice, salt, and pepper. Add the quinoa, tomatoes, spring onions (scallions), cucumber, olives, and herbs. Toss all of the ingredients in the dressing until they are thoroughly coated. Chill in the fridge for 1 hour before serving.

Smoked Mackerel & Cannellini Bean Salad

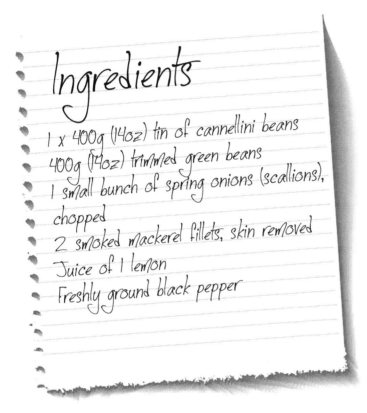

Ingredients

- 1 x 400g (14oz) tin of cannellini beans
- 400g (14oz) trimmed green beans
- 1 small bunch of spring onions (scallions), chopped
- 2 smoked mackerel fillets, skin removed
- Juice of 1 lemon
- Freshly ground black pepper

SERVES 2

Method

Slice the green beans in half and steam them for 4 minutes, or until they soften but maintain their crunch. Mix the green beans in a bowl together with the cannellini beans and chopped spring onions (scallions). Chop the mackerel fillets into small pieces and add to the bean mixture. Squeeze in the lemon juice and stir. Season with black pepper and serve.

Potato Salad

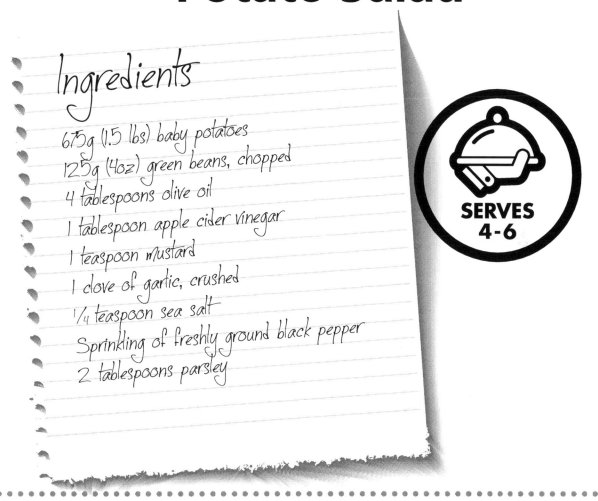

Ingredients

675g (1.5 lbs) baby potatoes
125g (4oz) green beans, chopped
4 tablespoons olive oil
1 tablespoon apple cider vinegar
1 teaspoon mustard
1 clove of garlic, crushed
1/4 teaspoon sea salt
Sprinkling of freshly ground black pepper
2 tablespoons parsley

SERVES 4-6

Method

Boil the potatoes for around 20 minutes or until they are cooked through. Drain and set aside. Steam the beans until they are tender. Place the olive oil, vinegar, mustard, garlic, salt and pepper in a bowl. Mix well. Once the potatoes and beans have cooled, add them to the bowl and coat in the dressing. Sprinkle with parsley and refrigerate before serving.

Mango & Avocado Salad

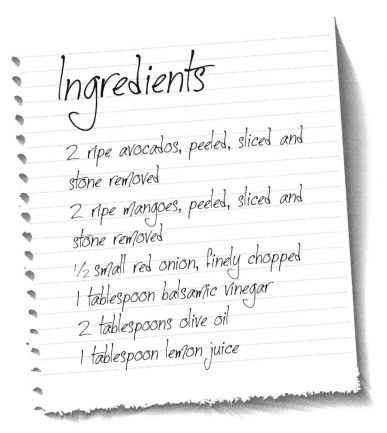

Ingredients

2 ripe avocados, peeled, sliced and stone removed

2 ripe mangoes, peeled, sliced and stone removed

½ small red onion, finely chopped

1 tablespoon balsamic vinegar

2 tablespoons olive oil

1 tablespoon lemon juice

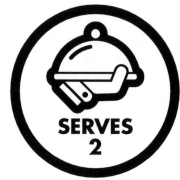

SERVES
2

Method

Mix together the balsamic vinegar, olive oil and lemon juice in a bowl. Add in the avocados, mango and onion. Stir and coat them with the dressing. Serve and eat immediately.

Beetroot & Orange Salad

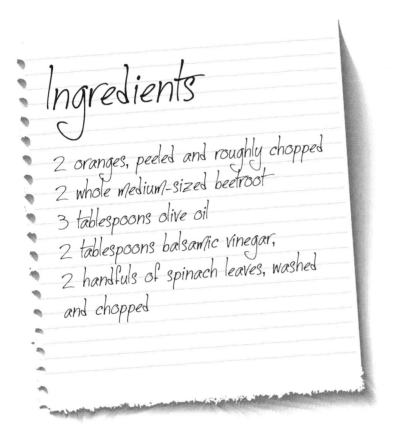

Ingredients

2 oranges, peeled and roughly chopped
2 whole medium-sized beetroot
3 tablespoons olive oil
2 tablespoons balsamic vinegar,
2 handfuls of spinach leaves, washed
and chopped

SERVES
4

Method

Place the whole beetroot on a baking tray and coat with a tablespoon of olive oil. Bake in the oven at 200C/400F for 45 minutes. Allow to cool. Peel and dice the beetroot. Place it in a bowl with the orange pieces and spinach leaves. In a cup, mix together 2 tablespoons of olive oil and balsamic vinegar. Pour the dressing over the salad before serving.

Lentil Curry

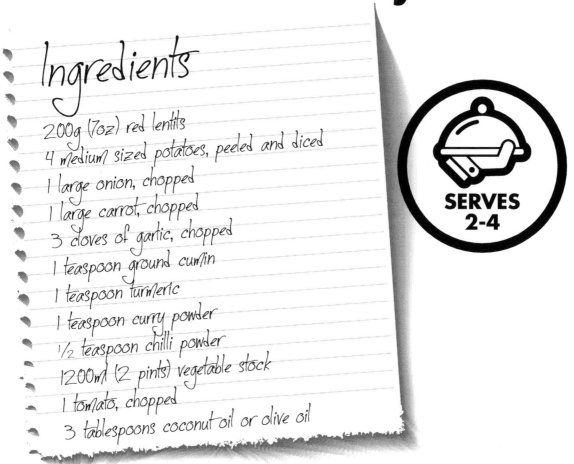

Ingredients

200g (7oz) red lentils
4 medium sized potatoes, peeled and diced
1 large onion, chopped
1 large carrot, chopped
3 cloves of garlic, chopped
1 teaspoon ground cumin
1 teaspoon turmeric
1 teaspoon curry powder
½ teaspoon chilli powder
1200ml (2 pints) vegetable stock
1 tomato, chopped
3 tablespoons coconut oil or olive oil

SERVES 2-4

Method

Heat the oil in a saucepan. Add the onion, tomato and garlic and cook for 5 minutes until the onion softens. Add the cumin, turmeric, curry powder and chilli and stir for 2 minutes. Add the carrots, potatoes, lentils and stock (broth). Bring to the boil, reduce the heat and simmer for 25-30 minutes. Serve with rice.

Bacon & Sweet Potato Hash

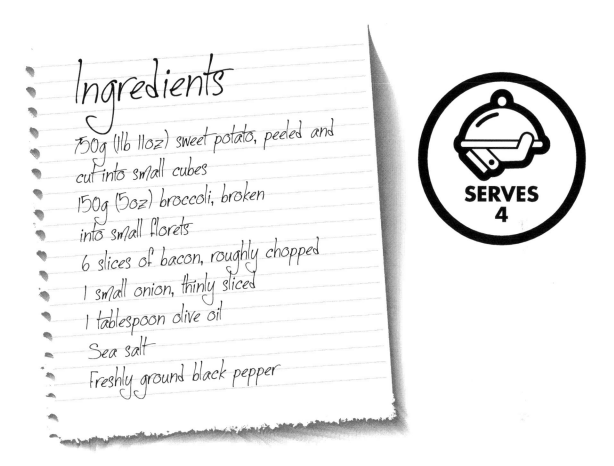

Ingredients

750g (1lb 11oz) sweet potato, peeled and
cut into small cubes

150g (5oz) broccoli, broken
into small florets

6 slices of bacon, roughly chopped

1 small onion, thinly sliced

1 tablespoon olive oil

Sea salt

Freshly ground black pepper

SERVES 4

Method

Steam the sweet potato for 10 minutes. Add the broccoli to the steamer and cook for
another 4 minutes. Heat the olive oil in a frying pan and add the bacon and onion. Fry for
5 minutes until the onion has softened and the bacon is cooked. Add the sweet potato
and broccoli to the pan and stir. Season with salt and pepper. Cook for around 10 minutes,
stirring to incorporate the crispy bits forming at the bottom.

Cauliflower Hash Browns

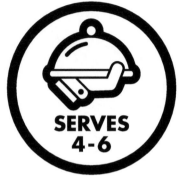

SERVES 4-6

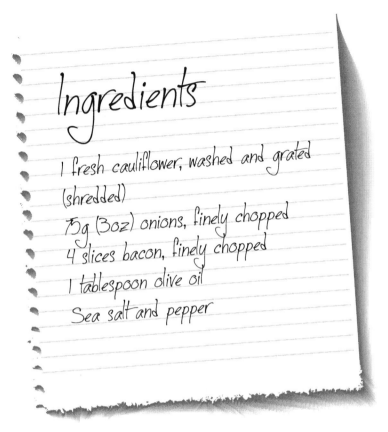

Ingredients

1 fresh cauliflower, washed and grated (shredded)

75g (3oz) onions, finely chopped

4 slices bacon, finely chopped

1 tablespoon olive oil

Sea salt and pepper

Method

Heat the oil in a frying pan and add the bacon and onion. Fry until the bacon starts to brown and the onion softens. Add the grated cauliflower. Stir and fry it until it is tender and golden brown. Add some extra olive oil if you need to. Season with salt and pepper and serve.

Gammon & Pineapple Salsa

Ingredients

4 gammon steaks
½ fresh ripe pineapple, diced finely
½ red onion, finely chopped
2.5cm (1 inch) chunk of fresh ginger, peel and finely chopped
1 teaspoon paprika
1 tablespoon fresh coriander (cilantro) leaves or mint, finely chopped
2 tablespoons olive oil

SERVES
4

Method

Place the pineapple, onion, ginger, paprika and coriander into a bowl with 1 tablespoon of olive oil and mix. Make several incisions in the gammon fat to prevent it curling up during cooking. Heat a tablespoon olive oil in a frying pan, add the gammon steaks and cook for 5-6 minutes on each side until slightly golden. Serve immediately with pineapple salsa on the side.

Florentine Pizza

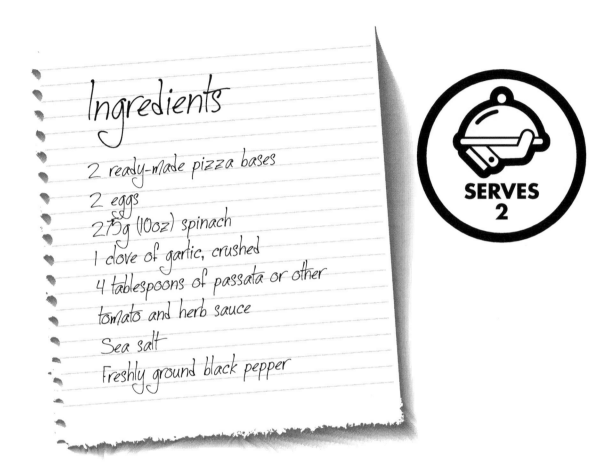

Ingredients

2 ready-made pizza bases

2 eggs

275g (10oz) spinach

1 clove of garlic, crushed

4 tablespoons of passata or other tomato and herb sauce

Sea salt

Freshly ground black pepper

SERVES 2

Method

Steam the spinach for 3-4 minutes. Drain and set aside to cool down then chop it roughly and mix with the garlic, salt and pepper. Divide the tomato sauce between the pizza bases and spread it evenly. Add the spinach and make a well in the middle ready to hold the egg. Bake the bases in the oven at 220C/425F for 5 minutes. Remove them from the oven and crack an egg into the well in the middle of the spinach. Return the pizza's to the oven and bake for 9-10 minutes until the eggs are set and the pizza bases are nice and crispy.

DINNER

Lamb Shanks with Lentils

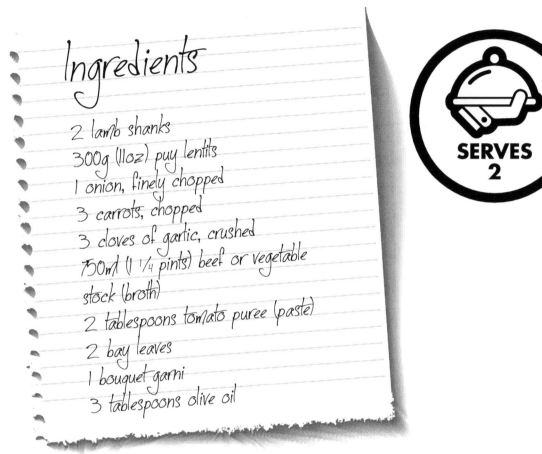

Ingredients

2 lamb shanks
300g (11oz) puy lentils
1 onion, finely chopped
3 carrots, chopped
3 cloves of garlic, crushed
750ml (1 1/4 pints) beef or vegetable stock (broth)
2 tablespoons tomato puree (paste)
2 bay leaves
1 bouquet garni
3 tablespoons olive oil

SERVES 2

Method

Place the oil in a large oven-proof casserole dish, place it on a hob at a high heat. Add the lamb, turning occasionally until it is brown all over. Transfer the lamb to a bowl and set aside. Add the onion, carrots and garlic to the casserole dish and cook for 5 minutes. Return the lamb to the dish and add in the stock, tomato puree (paste), bouquet garni, bay leaves and lentils. Cover the dish and transfer it to the oven. Cook at 200C/400F for 2 hours. Check half way through cooking and add extra stock (broth) or water if required. Serve and enjoy.

Prawn & Salmon Kebabs

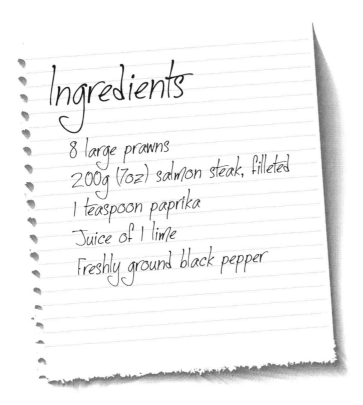

Ingredients

8 large prawns
200g (7oz) salmon steak, filleted
1 teaspoon paprika
Juice of 1 lime
Freshly ground black pepper

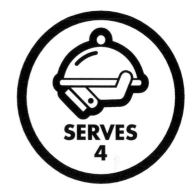

SERVES
4

Method

Remove the skin from the salmon. Cut it into chunks and place in a bowl. Add in the prawns. Cover with paprika, lime juice, and black pepper. Once the fish and prawns are coated, slide alternating pieces of salmon and prawns onto skewers. Place the kebabs under a hot grill (broiler) and cook for 3-4 minutes on each side, until cooked through.

Chicken & Red Pepper Risotto

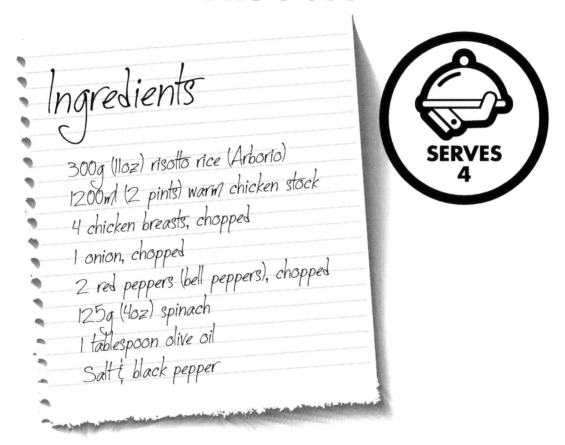

SERVES 4

Ingredients

300g (11oz) risotto rice (Arborio)

1200ml (2 pints) warm chicken stock

4 chicken breasts, chopped

1 onion, chopped

2 red peppers (bell peppers), chopped

125g (4oz) spinach

1 tablespoon olive oil

Salt & black pepper

Method

Heat the olive oil and a saucepan. Add the chicken, onion and red pepper (bell pepper). Cook for around 5-6 minutes. Add the rice to the pan, stir and cook for 2 minutes, until the rice is coated in oil. Slowly add the stock (broth) while stirring and adding a little at a time until all the liquid has been absorbed, around 15 minutes. Add the spinach to the pan. Cook for around 2 minutes, or until the spinach has wilted. Season and serve.

Lamb With Rosemary & Peppers

Ingredients

SERVES 4

1 onion, finely chopped
2 cloves of garlic, finely chopped
4 tablespoons olive oil
550g (1 1/4lb) lamb steaks, cubed
1 yellow pepper (bell pepper), sliced
1 red pepper (bell pepper), sliced
1 x 400g (14oz) tin of tomatoes
3 stalks of rosemary
Freshly ground black pepper

Method

Heat the oil in a saucepan and add the garlic and onion. Cook for 5 minutes until the onion softens. Remove the onion and garlic then set aside. Add the chopped lamb to the oil in the pan. Cook until golden brown. Remove and set aside. Return the onion and garlic to the pan and add the tomatoes, peppers and rosemary. Bring to the boil then reduce the heat and simmer for 10 minutes. Return the lamb to the pan and simmer for another 5-10 minutes. Season with black pepper. Remove the rosemary stalks and serve with sautéed potatoes or mash.

Ham & Turkey Rolls

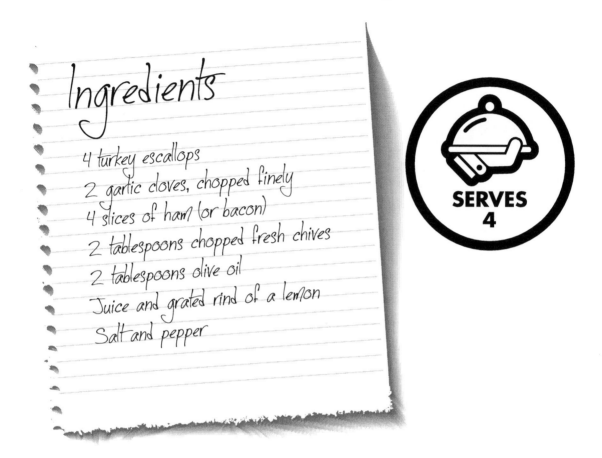

Ingredients

4 turkey escallops
2 garlic cloves, chopped finely
4 slices of ham (or bacon)
2 tablespoons chopped fresh chives
2 tablespoons olive oil
Juice and grated rind of a lemon
Salt and pepper

SERVES 4

Method

Halve each turkey escalope horizontally and spread it out. Season the inside with salt and pepper, then sprinkle with garlic, lemon juice, lemon rind and chopped chives. Join the two pieces together again. Roll each piece of turkey in a slice of ham. Secure them with wooden cocktail sticks. Heat the olive oil in a frying pan. Add the turkey rolls and cook for 4-5 minutes until they are golden brown. Turn over and coat with any remaining lemon juice. Cook for 3-4 minutes or until cooked through.

Chicken Fried Rice

Ingredients

200g (7oz) cooked chicken, cubed (leftovers are perfect for this)
225g (8oz) mushrooms, chopped
350g (12oz) rice, cooked
2 tablespoons soy sauce
2 eggs, beaten
4 spring onions (scallions)
2 tablespoons olive oil or coconut oil
3 cloves garlic, crushed

SERVES 2

Method

Heat a tablespoon of olive oil in a frying pan. Add the spring onions (scallions), and garlic and cook until they become soft. Transfer to a bowl and set aside. Add another tablespoon of olive oil to the pan. Pour in the eggs, stir until scrambled and firm. Place the eggs in a bowl and set aside. Then add the chicken, mushrooms, soy sauce, and cooked rice. Heat thoroughly. Add the cooked spring onions, garlic and eggs. Mix together then season and serve.

Cajun Salmon

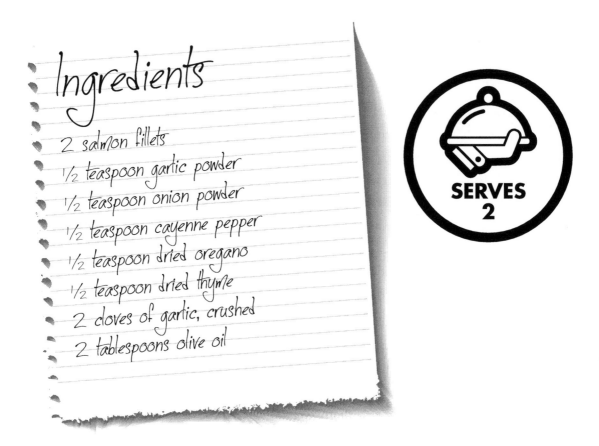

Ingredients

- 2 salmon fillets
- 1/2 teaspoon garlic powder
- 1/2 teaspoon onion powder
- 1/2 teaspoon cayenne pepper
- 1/2 teaspoon dried oregano
- 1/2 teaspoon dried thyme
- 2 cloves of garlic, crushed
- 2 tablespoons olive oil

SERVES 2

Method

Mix the spices together in a bowl. Sprinkle the skinless side of the salmon with the Cajun seasoning. Heat the olive oil in a frying pan and add the salmon, skin side down. Cook for 4 to 5 minutes on each side, turning gently. Remove and place the salmon fillets onto a serving plate. Stir the garlic into the oil in the pan. Cook for a minute or so and then pour all the garlic oil over the salmon.

Dairy Free Diet

Thyme & Garlic Roast Chicken

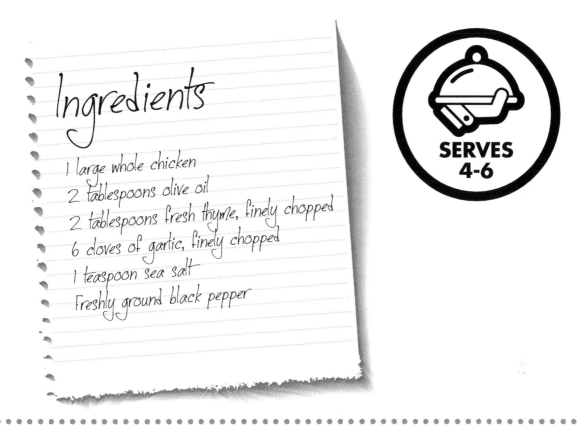

SERVES 4-6

Ingredients

1 large whole chicken
2 tablespoons olive oil
2 tablespoons fresh thyme, finely chopped
6 cloves of garlic, finely chopped
1 teaspoon sea salt
Freshly ground black pepper

Method

Place a tablespoon of oil, the garlic, thyme and salt in a small bowl and combine. Make an opening at the neck of the chicken and tuck the herb mixture under the skin. If you loosen the skin around the drumsticks you can press it in. Sprinkle with pepper. Place the chicken in an ovenproof dish, with a tablespoon of olive oil. Roast in the oven at 180C/350F for around 1½ hours, basting with the cooking juices. Test with a skewer and when the juices run clear, remove from the oven. Allow the chicken to stand for a few minutes before serving.

Nasi Goreng (Indonesian Fried Rice)

Ingredients

250g (9 oz) rice
2 tablespoons thai red curry paste
250g (9 oz) pork steaks, cut into strips
200g (7oz) frozen cooked prawns, defrosted
1 tablespoon soy sauce (tamari soy sauce
if gluten-free)
200g (7oz) frozen peas, defrosted
2 eggs, whisked
2 tablespoons fresh coriander, chopped

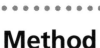

SERVES 4

Method

Cook the rice according to the instructions on the packet then set aside. Heat the curry paste and add the pork strips. Cook for 5 minutes until thoroughly cooked. Add the prawns, peas, soy sauce and cooked rice. Fry for 5-6 minutes. Move the rice mixture to one side of the pan. In the clear part of the pan add the beaten eggs. Cook until they become firm before mixing with the rest of the ingredients. Sprinkle in the chopped coriander. Serve and enjoy.

Chilli Beef, Asparagus & Corn

Ingredients

2 tablespoons groundnut oil
300g (11oz) beef strips, or steak cut into thin strips
200g (7oz) baby corn
200g (7oz) asparagus, chopped
1 small onion, sliced
2 red chillies, deseeded and finely sliced
2 cloves of garlic, crushed
2 tablespoons soy sauce
Juice of ½ a lime

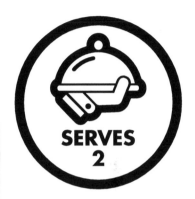

SERVES 2

Method

Heat the oil in a wok or large frying pan. Add the garlic and chilli. Cook for 30 seconds. Add the baby corn, onion and asparagus and cook for 3 minutes. Add the beef and fry for 2-3 minutes or until the meat is lightly browned. Add the lime juice and soy sauce. Cook until heated through and serve with rice and salad.

Cottage Pie

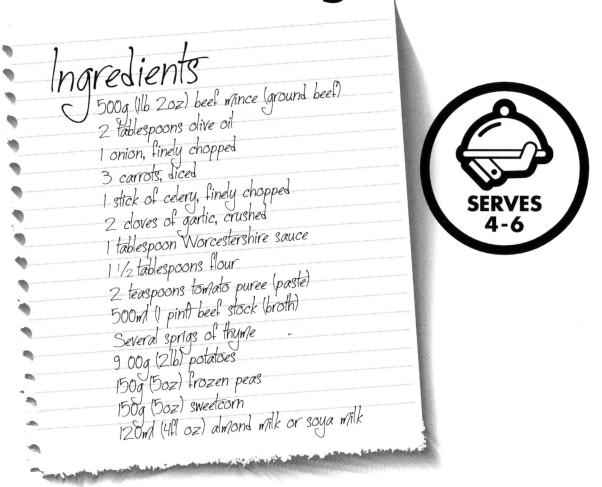

Ingredients

- 500g (1lb 2oz) beef mince (ground beef)
- 2 tablespoons olive oil
- 1 onion, finely chopped
- 3 carrots, diced
- 1 stick of celery, finely chopped
- 2 cloves of garlic, crushed
- 1 tablespoon Worcestershire sauce
- 1½ tablespoons flour
- 2 teaspoons tomato puree (paste)
- 500ml (1 pint) beef stock (broth)
- Several sprigs of thyme
- 900g (2lb) potatoes
- 150g (5oz) frozen peas
- 150g (5oz) sweetcorn
- 120ml (4fl oz) almond milk or soya milk

SERVES 4-6

Method

Heat a tablespoon of oil in a saucepan, add the beef and cook until brown. Remove it from the pan and set aside. Put another tablespoon of oil into the pan and add the onion, carrots, celery and garlic. Reduce the heat and cook for 15 minutes. Add the tomato puree and flour and stir. Return the beef to the pan and add the Worcestershire sauce, stock (broth), and thyme. Simmer uncovered for 30 minutes to reduce the gravy. Add the peas and sweetcorn to the meat. In the meantime, boil the potatoes until tender. Drain off the water and mash the potatoes, adding in the almond or soya milk. Season with salt and pepper. Spoon the meat into a casserole dish or individual pie dishes. Cover the meat with mashed potato. Bake in the oven at 220C/400F for 20 minutes or until the top of the pie is golden.

Fish Pie

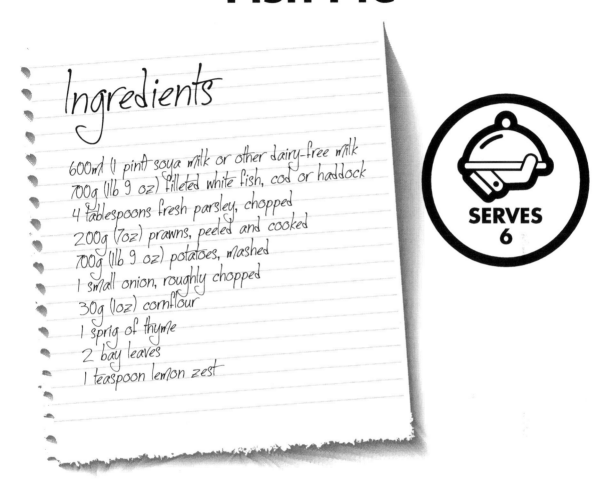

Ingredients

600ml (1 pint) soya milk or other dairy-free milk
700g (1lb 9 oz) filleted white fish, cod or haddock
4 tablespoons fresh parsley, chopped
200g (7oz) prawns, peeled and cooked
700g (1lb 9 oz) potatoes, mashed
1 small onion, roughly chopped
30g (1oz) cornflour
1 sprig of thyme
2 bay leaves
1 teaspoon lemon zest

SERVES 6

Method

Place the soya or other dairy-free milk in a saucepan with the onion, bay leaves, thyme and lemon zest. Add the fish and bring to the boil. Gently simmer for 15 minutes until the fish is cooked through. Strain the milk off the fish and set aside, ready to make the sauce. Discard the onion, bay leaves, thyme and zest. Flake the fish into chunks and place in an oven-proof casserole dish. To make the sauce, mix the cornflour with enough water or dairy-free milk to make a paste. Stir the paste into the milk you set aside. Place it on the heat and stir until it thickens. Add in the parsley and prawns. Stir and cook for 2 minutes. Pour the sauce over the fish. Top it off with mashed potatoes. Transfer the fish pie to the oven and cook for 30 minutes at 180C/350F until the mashed potato is slightly golden.

Pork, Pine Nuts & Basil

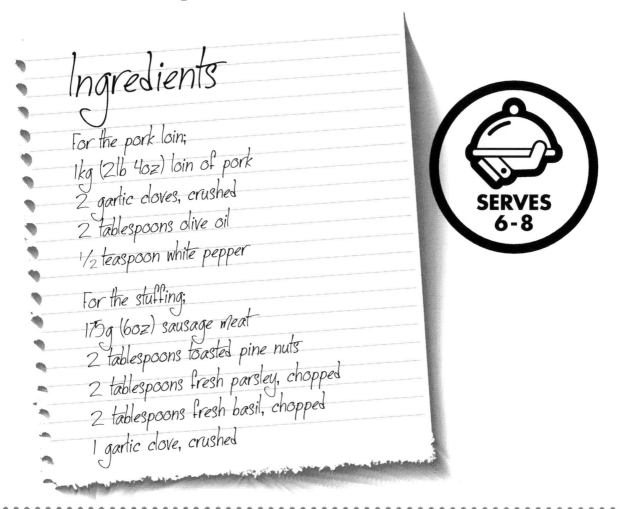

Ingredients

For the pork loin;

1kg (2lb 4oz) loin of pork
2 garlic cloves, crushed
2 tablespoons olive oil
1/2 teaspoon white pepper

For the stuffing;

175g (6oz) sausage meat
2 tablespoons toasted pine nuts
2 tablespoons fresh parsley, chopped
2 tablespoons fresh basil, chopped
1 garlic clove, crushed

SERVES 6-8

Method

Lay out the pork and make a long cut lengthwise, stopping around 2 cm (1 inch) from the edge of the meat, creating a crevice for the stuffing. Rub the 2 cloves of garlic and pepper all over the pork. In a bowl, combine the sausage meat, pine nuts, parsley, basil and garlic. Stuff the sausage mixture into the incision in the pork. Pull the two sides of the pork loin together and wrap it in foil, twisting the foil at the end. Chill for 1 hour.

Heat the olive oil in a pan. Unwrap the pork loin and cook in the pan for 4 minutes, turning once. Transfer to an ovenproof dish, place in the oven and cook at 180C/350F for 35 minutes. Remove, slice it and serve.

Garlic Mushrooms & Prawns

SERVES 4

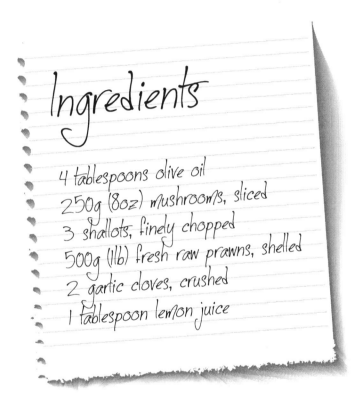

Ingredients

4 tablespoons olive oil
250g (8oz) mushrooms, sliced
3 shallots, finely chopped
500g (1lb) fresh raw prawns, shelled
2 garlic cloves, crushed
1 tablespoon lemon juice

Method

Heat the oil in a large frying pan. Add the garlic, shallots and mushrooms and fry until they soften. Add the prawns, and cook until they are pink throughout. Add the lemon juice and cook for another minute. Season and serve with rice, couscous or salad.

Pork Escalopes & Red Wine

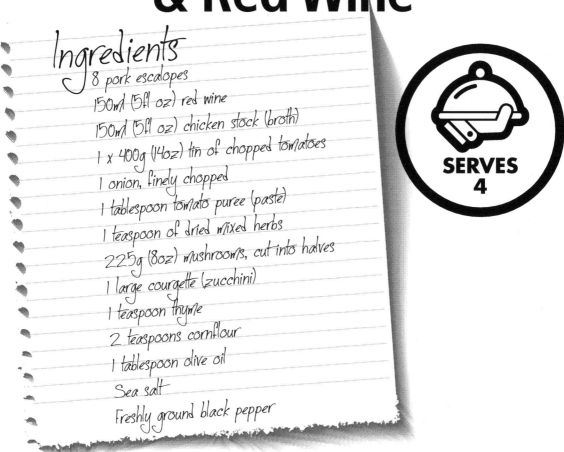

Ingredients

8 pork escalopes

150ml (5fl oz) red wine

150ml (5fl oz) chicken stock (broth)

1 x 400g (14oz) tin of chopped tomatoes

1 onion, finely chopped

1 tablespoon tomato puree (paste)

1 teaspoon of dried mixed herbs

225g (8oz) mushrooms, cut into halves

1 large courgette (zucchini)

1 teaspoon thyme

2 teaspoons cornflour

1 tablespoon olive oil

Sea salt

Freshly ground black pepper

SERVES 4

Method

Heat the oil in a frying pan and cook the pork and onions for 5 minutes. Add in the tomatoes, tomato puree, red wine, herbs, stock (broth) courgette, and mushrooms. Cover and simmer for 15 minutes. Mix together the cornflour with 2 tablespoons water to form a smooth paste. Stir the cornflour mixture into the pan. Stir and simmer for 2 minutes until the sauce thickens. Season with salt and pepper before serving.

Chicken Chasseur

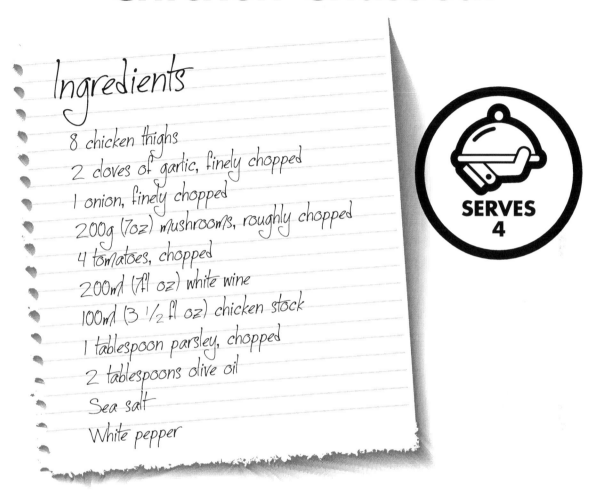

Ingredients

8 chicken thighs
2 cloves of garlic, finely chopped
1 onion, finely chopped
200g (7oz) mushrooms, roughly chopped
4 tomatoes, chopped
200ml (7fl oz) white wine
100ml (3 ½ fl oz) chicken stock
1 tablespoon parsley, chopped
2 tablespoons olive oil
Sea salt
White pepper

SERVES 4

Method

Heat a tablespoon of oil in a pan and add the chicken. Season it with salt and pepper. Cook for 2 minutes on each side. Remove the chicken and keep it warm. Add a tablespoon of olive oil to the pan and add the garlic, onions, tomatoes and the mushrooms. Sauté for 5 minutes. Return the chicken to the pan and add the stock (broth), white wine and parsley. Bring it to the boil, reduce the heat and simmer for 30 minutes.

Lamb Chops with Coriander & Lime

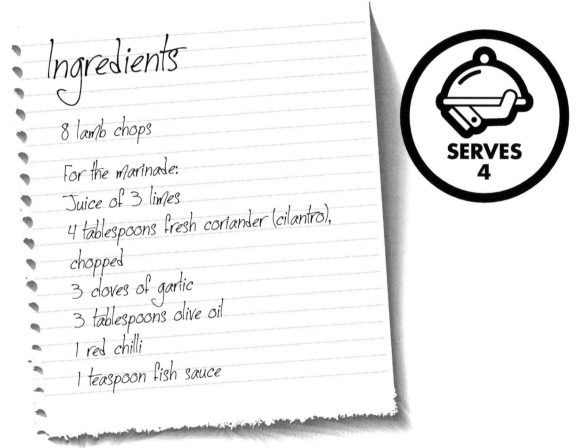

Ingredients

8 lamb chops

For the marinade:
Juice of 3 limes
4 tablespoons fresh coriander (cilantro), chopped
3 cloves of garlic
3 tablespoons olive oil
1 red chilli
1 teaspoon fish sauce

SERVES 4

Method

Place all the ingredients for the marinade into a blender and blitz until smooth. Transfer half of the marinade to a separate bowl to be used as a dressing after cooking. Put the lamb onto a plate and pour the other half of the dressing over the lamb. Marinate for 40 minutes. Grill the lamb chops for around 4 minutes on each side. Longer if you like them well cooked. Serve the chops onto plates and spoon over the dressing.

Beef Kebabs

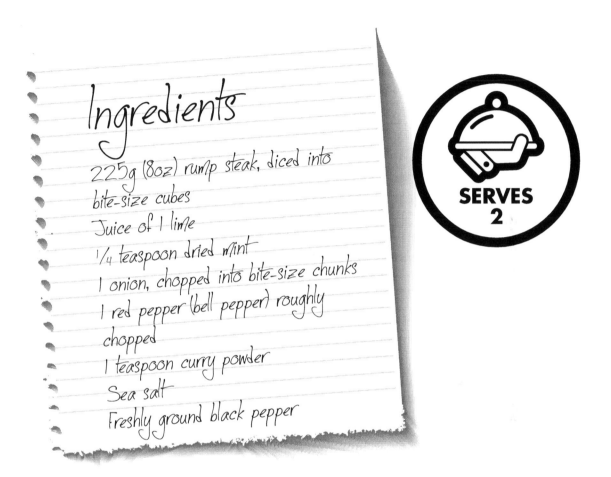

Ingredients

225g (8oz) rump steak, diced into
bite-size cubes
Juice of 1 lime
1/4 teaspoon dried mint
1 onion, chopped into bite-size chunks
1 red pepper (bell pepper) roughly
chopped
1 teaspoon curry powder
Sea salt
Freshly ground black pepper

**SERVES
2**

Method

Mix together the curry powder, lime juice, mint, salt and pepper in a bowl. Add the meat cubes, onion and red pepper. Stir to coat the ingredients with the curry mixture. Thread the meat, red pepper and onion onto skewers, alternating them as you go. Place under a preheated grill for 9-10 minutes turning during cooking ensure they're evenly cooked.

Chickpea and Vegetable Casserole

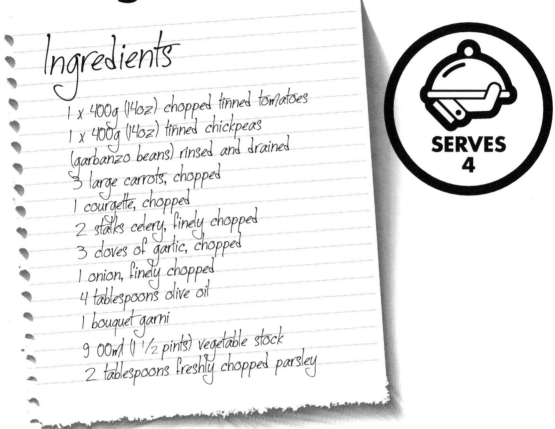

Ingredients

1 x 400g (14oz) chopped tinned tomatoes
1 x 400g (14oz) tinned chickpeas
(garbanzo beans) rinsed and drained
3 large carrots, chopped
1 courgette, chopped
2 stalks celery, finely chopped
3 cloves of garlic, chopped
1 onion, finely chopped
4 tablespoons olive oil
1 bouquet garni
900ml (1 ½ pints) vegetable stock
2 tablespoons freshly chopped parsley

SERVES 4

Method

Heat the oil in a saucepan and add the onion and garlic. Cook gently for 5 minutes. Add in the carrots, celery and tinned tomatoes. Cook for another 5 minutes. Add the chickpeas courgette, bouquet garni and stock (broth) to the saucepan. Simmer for 15 minutes. Sprinkle in the parsley and serve.

Beef, Green Pepper & Black Beans

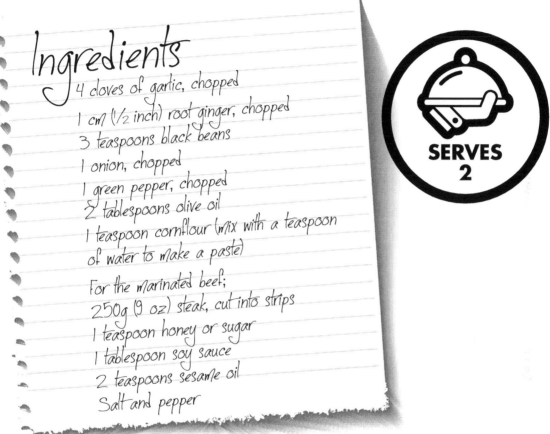

Ingredients

4 cloves of garlic, chopped

1 cm (½ inch) root ginger, chopped

3 teaspoons black beans

1 onion, chopped

1 green pepper, chopped

2 tablespoons olive oil

1 teaspoon cornflour (mix with a teaspoon of water to make a paste)

For the marinated beef;

250g (9 oz) steak, cut into strips

1 teaspoon honey or sugar

1 tablespoon soy sauce

2 teaspoons sesame oil

Salt and pepper

SERVES 2

Method

Combine the beef with the honey or sugar, soy sauce, sesame oil, salt and pepper and marinade for at least an hour. Mix together the ginger, garlic, and black beans with a tablespoon of olive oil then set aside. Heat a tablespoon of olive oil in a frying pan or wok. Add the meat and stir-fry for 3-4 minutes. Remove the meat and keep it warm. Put the green pepper and onion into the pan. Cook for 3 minutes then return the beef to the pan. Add in the ginger, garlic and black beans and cook for 2-3 minutes. Remove from the heat and stir in the cornflour paste. Stir until it thickens. Serve with rice and enjoy.

Spaghetti Bolognese

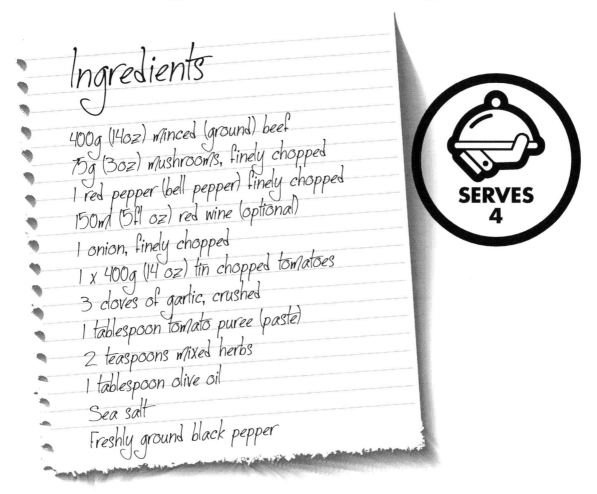

Ingredients

400g (14oz) minced (ground) beef
75g (3oz) mushrooms, finely chopped
1 red pepper (bell pepper) finely chopped
150ml (5fl oz) red wine (optional)
1 onion, finely chopped
1 x 400g (14 oz) tin chopped tomatoes
3 cloves of garlic, crushed
1 tablespoon tomato puree (paste)
2 teaspoons mixed herbs
1 tablespoon olive oil
Sea salt
Freshly ground black pepper

SERVES 4

Method

Heat the olive oil in a large saucepan and add the onion and garlic and cook until the onion softens. Add the red pepper (bell pepper), minced beef and cook until the meat browns. Pour in the red wine (optional) and add the mushrooms. Cook for 2-3 minutes. Pour in the tinned tomatoes, tomato puree and herbs. Simmer for 15-20 minutes. Season the Bolognese with salt and pepper. Serve onto a bed of spaghetti.

Turkey & Tarragon Risotto

Ingredients

1 tablespoon olive oil
2 turkey steaks, chopped
225g (8oz) risotto rice (Arborio)
1 onion, finely chopped
1 small leek, finely chopped
2 cloves of garlic, crushed
600ml (1 pint) chicken stock (broth)
1 tablespoon fresh parsley, finely chopped
1 tablespoon fresh tarragon, finely chopped

SERVES 2

Method

Heat the oil in a large pan and add the leek, onion and garlic. Cook for around 5 minutes until they have softened. Stir in the turkey and cook for 3 minutes. Add in the risotto rice, stirring until it's coated in oil. Pour in the stock (broth) a little at a time, allowing the liquid to be absorbed before adding any more. Cook until the rice is soft and tender. Sprinkle in the fresh herbs and mix well. Serve and eat immediately.

Ratatouille

Ingredients

- 2 courgettes (zucchini), chopped
- 1 aubergine, chopped
- 1 red onion, chopped
- 2 cloves of garlic, crushed
- 1 red pepper (bell pepper) chopped
- 1 x 400g (14oz) tin chopped tomatoes
- 100ml (3½ fl oz) red wine
- 1 tablespoon tomato puree (paste)
- 1 handful of fresh mixed herbs, oregano, basil, marjoram or thyme
- 3 tablespoons olive oil

SERVES 4

Method

Heat the olive oil in a saucepan and sauté the courgettes (zucchini) and aubergines for 5 minutes. Remove and set aside. Put the garlic, red pepper (bell pepper) and onion into the pan and cook for 5 minutes. Add the tomato puree, tinned tomatoes and red wine and mix well. Return the aubergines and courgettes to the pan. Cover and simmer gently for 15 minutes. Sprinkle with herbs then serve.

Ham & Pineapple Pizza

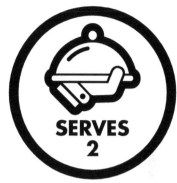

SERVES 2

Ingredients

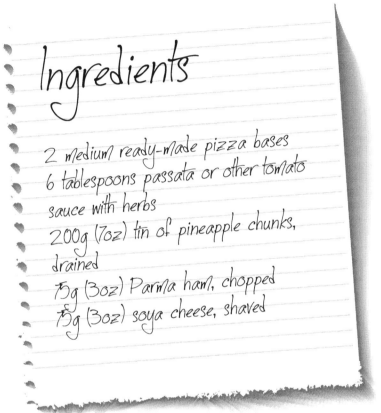

2 medium ready-made pizza bases
6 tablespoons passata or other tomato sauce with herbs
200g (7oz) tin of pineapple chunks, drained
75g (3oz) Parma ham, chopped
75g (3oz) soya cheese, shaved

Method

Spread the passata over the pizza bases and sprinkle with the pineapple chunks and the ham. Bake for 12 minutes until the base is starting to turn brown and the tomato sauce is bubbling. Remove the pizza from the oven and scatter the soya cheese over the top, then return to the oven for 3–4 minutes until the cheese has started to melt. Serve and eat immediately.

Mustard & Ginger Chicken

Ingredients

4 chicken breasts
1 tablespoon olive oil
2 red onions, finely chopped
2.5cm (1 inch) chunk of root ginger, crushed
2 cloves of garlic, crushed
300ml (10fl oz) chicken stock (broth)
1 teaspoon Tabasco sauce
1 teaspoon paprika
2 teaspoons mustard
1 teaspoon honey
Sea Salt
Freshly ground black pepper

SERVES 4

Method

Heat the olive oil in a frying pan and add the chicken breasts. Cook the chicken for 2 minutes on each side then remove them, cover and set aside. Add the onion, garlic and ginger to the pan and cook for 5 minutes until the onion softens. Add the stock (broth), mustard, paprika, Tabasco sauce and honey. Bring to the boil then reduce the heat. Return the chicken to the pan and simmer gently for 10 minutes. Season with salt and pepper before serving.

Caribbean Chicken

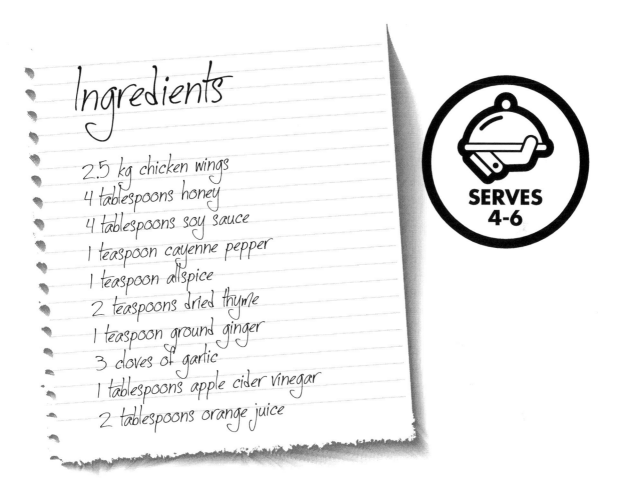

Ingredients

2.5 kg chicken wings
4 tablespoons honey
4 tablespoons soy sauce
1 teaspoon cayenne pepper
1 teaspoon allspice
2 teaspoons dried thyme
1 teaspoon ground ginger
3 cloves of garlic
1 tablespoons apple cider vinegar
2 tablespoons orange juice

SERVES 4-6

Method

Apart from the chicken, place all the other ingredients into a food processor. Blitz the ingredients until you have a smooth paste. Put the chicken in a large bowl and add the marinade. Stir coat the chicken completely. Transfer the chicken to 2 baking sheets and place in the oven. Roast the chicken wings at 180C/350F for 35-40 minutes. Can be served hot or cold.

Mushroom & Nut Loaf

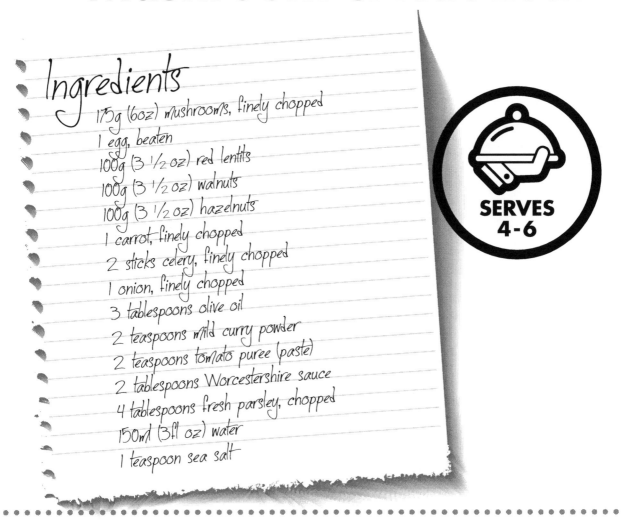

Ingredients

- 175g (6oz) mushrooms, finely chopped
- 1 egg, beaten
- 100g (3 ½ oz) red lentils
- 100g (3 ½ oz) walnuts
- 100g (3 ½ oz) hazelnuts
- 1 carrot, finely chopped
- 2 sticks celery, finely chopped
- 1 onion, finely chopped
- 3 tablespoons olive oil
- 2 teaspoons mild curry powder
- 2 teaspoons tomato puree (paste)
- 2 tablespoons Worcestershire sauce
- 4 tablespoons fresh parsley, chopped
- 150ml (3fl oz) water
- 1 teaspoon sea salt

SERVES 4-6

Method

Steep the lentils in cold water for 1 hour. Heat the olive oil in a pan and add the carrot, celery, onion, mushrooms and curry powder. Cook for 5 minutes. Blitz the nuts in a food processor and set aside. Drain the lentils, place them in a bowl and add the nuts. Stir in the cooked vegetables, tomato paste, Worcestershire sauce, egg, parsley, water and salt. Grease and line a large loaf tin with greaseproof paper. Put the mixture into the loaf tin and smooth it out. Cover with foil. Bake in the oven at 190C/375F for 60-90 minutes. Let it stand for 10 minutes then turn onto a serving plate.

Swordfish With Lemon & Basil

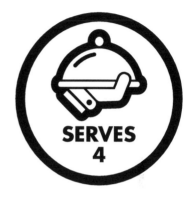

SERVES 4

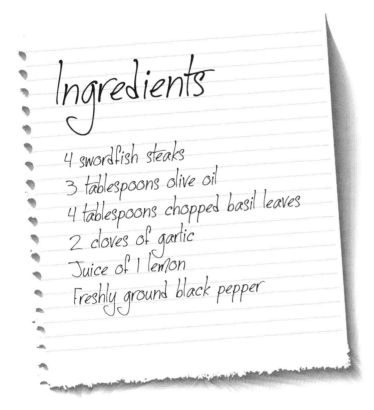

Ingredients

- 4 swordfish steaks
- 3 tablespoons olive oil
- 4 tablespoons chopped basil leaves
- 2 cloves of garlic
- Juice of 1 lemon
- Freshly ground black pepper

Method

Mix together the lemon juice, olive oil, garlic and basil and season with pepper. Place the fish on a plate and lightly coat the swordfish with 1-2 tablespoons of the lemon oil mixture. Heat a little olive oil in a hot pan and add the swordfish steaks. Cook for 3-4 minutes on each side and check that it's completely cooked. Serve onto plates with the remaining dressing.

Salmon Steaks & Tomato Salsa

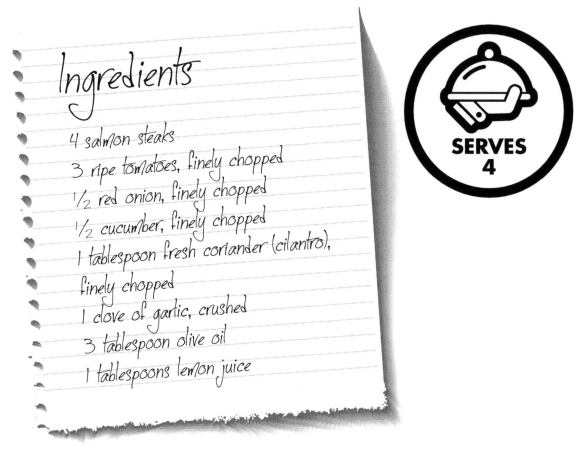

SERVES 4

Ingredients

4 salmon steaks

3 ripe tomatoes, finely chopped

1/2 red onion, finely chopped

1/2 cucumber, finely chopped

1 tablespoon fresh coriander (cilantro), finely chopped

1 clove of garlic, crushed

3 tablespoon olive oil

1 tablespoons lemon juice

Method

Place the tomatoes, onion, cucumber, garlic coriander (cilantro), lemon juice and 2 table-spoons of olive oil in a bowl and mix well. Set aside. Heat a tablespoon of olive oil in a frying pan. Add the salmon fillets and cook for 4-5 minutes on each side or until cooked thoroughly. Serve with the tomato salsa on the side.

Sea Bass with Green Vegetables

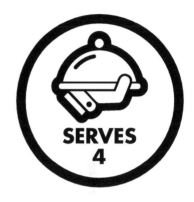

SERVES 4

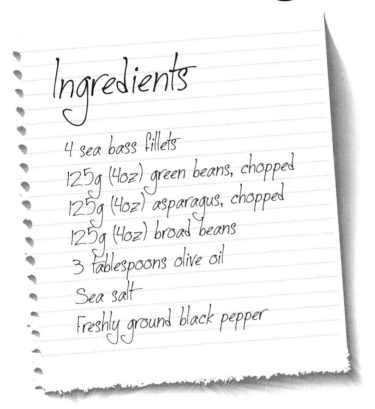

Ingredients

4 sea bass fillets
125g (4oz) green beans, chopped
125g (4oz) asparagus, chopped
125g (4oz) broad beans
3 tablespoons olive oil
Sea salt
Freshly ground black pepper

Method

Heat the olive oil in a pan then add the fish fillets. Season well with salt and pepper and fry them for around 3 minutes on each side. Meanwhile place the green beans, asparagus and broad beans into a steamer and cook for 5 minutes until cooked through but crisp. Season and serve them onto a plate and add the fish to the bed of vegetables. Enjoy.

Spicy Bean Burgers

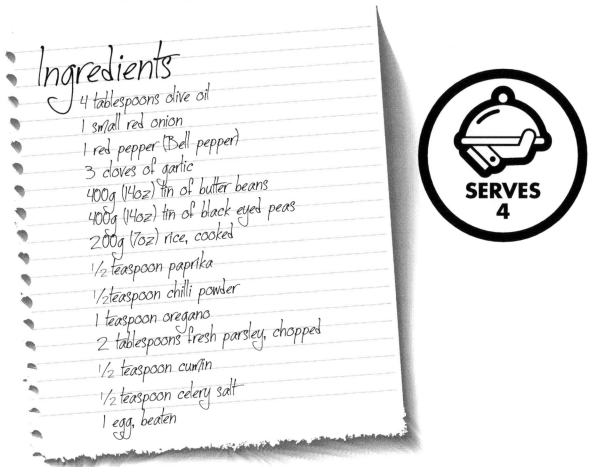

Ingredients
- 4 tablespoons olive oil
- 1 small red onion
- 1 red pepper (Bell pepper)
- 3 cloves of garlic
- 400g (14oz) tin of butter beans
- 400g (14oz) tin of black eyed peas
- 200g (7oz) rice, cooked
- 1/2 teaspoon paprika
- 1/2 teaspoon chilli powder
- 1 teaspoon oregano
- 2 tablespoons fresh parsley, chopped
- 1/2 teaspoon cumin
- 1/2 teaspoon celery salt
- 1 egg, beaten

SERVES 4

Method

Place the olive oil in a pan and add the onion, garlic and red pepper. Cook until they soften. Transfer them to a large bowl and add in the butterbeans and black eyed peas and rice. Add the paprika, chilli powder, oregano, parsley, cumin, celery salt and the beaten egg. Form the mixture into burger shapes. Fry the burgers for 3-4 minutes on each side. Serve and enjoy.

Thai Green Curry

Ingredients

4 chicken breasts, cut into bite-size chunks
2 stalks of lemon grass (inner stalks only)
400ml (14fl oz) coconut milk
75g (3oz) green beans, sliced
1 green chilli, de-seeded and chopped
4 tablespoons fresh coriander (cilantro),
chopped
2 tablespoons Thai green curry paste
2 teaspoons coconut oil
4 tablespoons basil leaves, torn
1 tablespoon fish sauce
Juice of a lime

SERVES 4

Method

Heat the coconut oil in a pan and add the green curry paste. Cook for 2-3 minutes. Depending on how tough the lemon grass is, either bruise the stalk to release flavour or finely chop the soft inner stalks. Add the coconut milk and lemongrass and simmer for 5 minutes. Add the chicken, coriander, green beans, and chilli. Bring to the boil, reduce the heat and simmer gently for 15 minutes. Stir in the fish sauce, basil and add the lime juice. Cook for another 2 minutes. You may wish to remove large pieces of lemongrass. Serve with brown rice.

Sausage Casserole

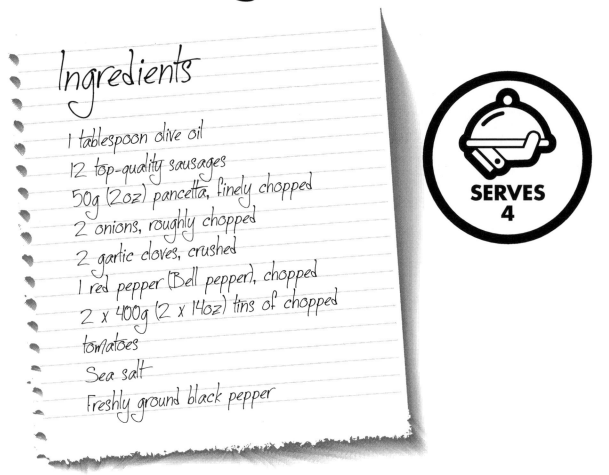

Ingredients

1 tablespoon olive oil
12 top-quality sausages
50g (2oz) pancetta, finely chopped
2 onions, roughly chopped
2 garlic cloves, crushed
1 red pepper (Bell pepper), chopped
2 x 400g (2 x 14oz) tins of chopped
tomatoes
Sea salt
Freshly ground black pepper

SERVES 4

Method

Heat the oil in a pan, add the sausages and pancetta and fry for 10 minutes until the sausages are nicely golden and the pancetta is crispy. Remove and set aside. Remove the excess fat. Put the onions and garlic in the pan and cook for 4 minutes then add the chopped red pepper and fry for another 2 minutes. Add the sausages and pancetta to the pan and stir in the chopped tomatoes. Cover the pan and cook on a medium heat for 20 minutes. Season with salt and pepper and serve.

Braised Beef & Mushrooms

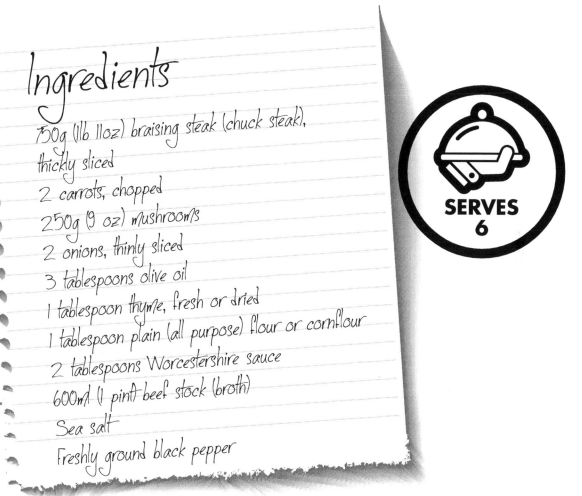

Ingredients

750g (1lb 11oz) braising steak (chuck steak),
thickly sliced
2 carrots, chopped
250g (9 oz) mushrooms
2 onions, thinly sliced
3 tablespoons olive oil
1 tablespoon thyme, fresh or dried
1 tablespoon plain (all purpose) flour or cornflour
2 tablespoons Worcestershire sauce
600ml (1 pint) beef stock (broth)
Sea salt
Freshly ground black pepper

SERVES 6

Method

Coat the beef with flour and season with salt and pepper. Heat the olive oil in a pan, then add the meat and brown it for 4 minutes. Remove the meat from the pan and set aside. Add to the pan the onions and fry until softened. Place the onions and meat in an oven-proof casserole dish. Add the mushrooms, carrots, beef stock (broth) Worcestershire sauce and thyme. Season and cover. Cook in the oven at 150C/300F for 1½-2 hours until the meat is tender.

DESSERTS, PUDDINGS & SNACKS

Coconut Macaroons

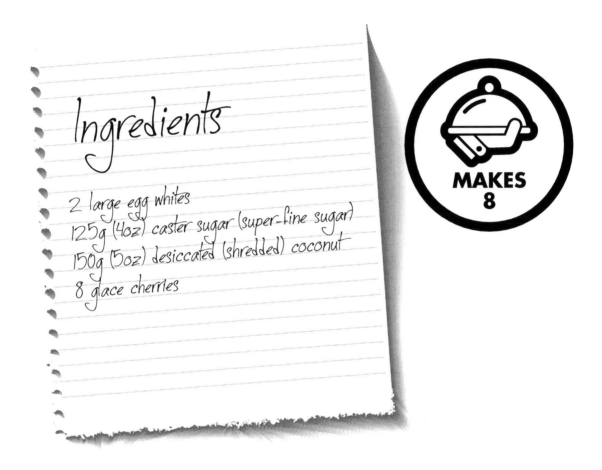

Ingredients

2 large egg whites
125g (4oz) caster sugar (super-fine sugar)
150g (5oz) desiccated (shredded) coconut
8 glace cherries

MAKES
8

Method

Grease and line a baking sheet. Place the separated egg whites in a bowl and whisk into soft peaks. Add in the sugar using a metal spoon and fold until all the sugar is mixed in. Combine with the coconut. Spoon the mixture onto the baking sheet, making 8 large rounded shapes. Place a glace cherry on top of each one. Transfer to the oven and bake at 180C/350F for 15-20 minutes until golden. Allow to cool for 5 minutes then transfer them to a wire rack.

Raspberry & Blueberry Low-Carb Crumble

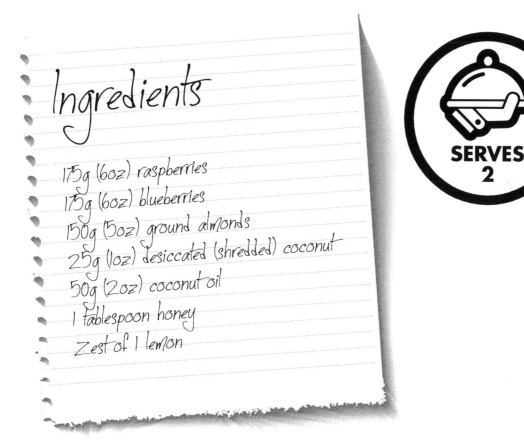

Ingredients

- 175g (6oz) raspberries
- 175g (6oz) blueberries
- 150g (5oz) ground almonds
- 25g (1oz) desiccated (shredded) coconut
- 50g (2oz) coconut oil
- 1 tablespoon honey
- Zest of 1 lemon

SERVES 2

Method

Place the ground almonds, coconut and lemon zest in a bowl and mix together. Warm the honey and coconut oil and pour into the almond mixture and combine. Put the raspberries and blueberries into an ovenproof dish. Cover them with the almond and coconut mixture. Bake in the oven at 180C/350F for 15 minutes until the top becomes slightly golden.

Spiced Poached Peaches

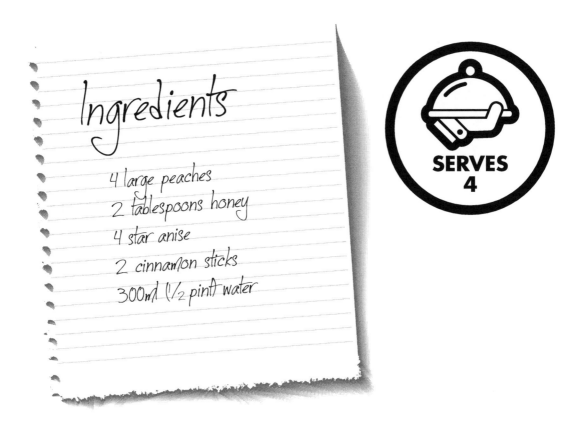

Ingredients

4 large peaches
2 tablespoons honey
4 star anise
2 cinnamon sticks
300ml (1/2 pint) water

SERVES
4

Method

Place the honey and water in a saucepan and bring to the boil. Add the peaches, star anise and cinnamon sticks. Reduce the heat and simmer gently for 10 minutes. Remove the peaches and set aside. Continue cooking the liquid for another 12-14 minutes until it begins to thicken. If necessary, return the peaches to the saucepan to warm them before serving.

Chocolate Ice Cream

Ingredients
1 x 400ml (14fl oz) tin coconut milk (full fat)
2 ripe bananas
3 tablespoons of 100% cocoa powder
2 tablespoons honey (optional) or a little stevia sweetener

SERVES
2

Method

Place the bananas, coconut milk and cocoa powder into a blender. Blitz until smooth. The ice cream is already sweet with the banana, however taste it and add honey or stevia if you wish to make it sweeter. Transfer it to an ice cream maker and process it for the required time depending on your machine. Freeze or eat straight away.

Strawberry Ice Cream

Ingredients
2 x 400ml (2 x 14fl oz) tins of coconut milk
450g (1lb) strawberries
2 tablespoons honey (optional) or a little stevia sweetener

SERVES
4

Method

Place the coconut milk and strawberries into a blender and blitz until smooth. Taste the cream for sweetness and add honey or sweetener if required. Transfer to an ice cream maker and process according to your manufacturer's instructions.

Crème Caramel

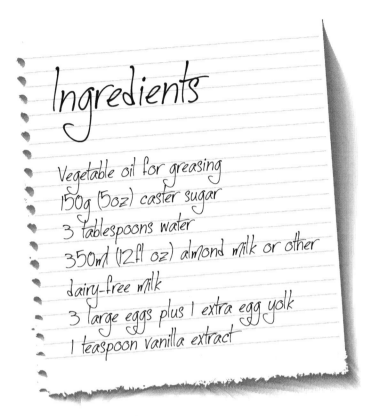

Ingredients

Vegetable oil for greasing
150g (5oz) caster sugar
3 tablespoons water
350ml (12fl oz) almond milk or other dairy-free milk
3 large eggs plus 1 extra egg yolk
1 teaspoon vanilla extract

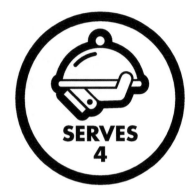

SERVES
4

Method

Grease four ramekins with a little vegetable oil. Put 125g (4oz) sugar into a saucepan and add the 3 tablespoons of water. Heat gently for 6–8 minutes until the sugar has caramelised taking care not to burn it. Pour the caramel into the ramekins. Use a mixer to beat together the eggs, extra egg yolk and the vanilla extract with the remaining sugar. Mix it until thick and smooth. Pour the almond milk into a saucepan and bring to the boil. Remove from the heat and slowly add the almond milk to the egg mixture and mix thoroughly.

Divide the milk mixture into the individual ramekins and put them in a roasting dish. Pour enough boiling water into the roasting dish to come halfway up the sides of the ramekins. Bake at 150C/300F for 30–35 minutes until set firm and golden. Remove from the oven and leave to cool. Cover and leave to chill in the fridge for 10-12 hours. Serve chilled.

Brownies

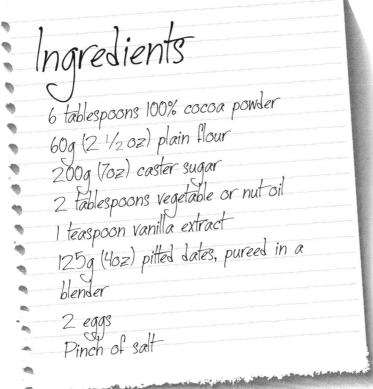

Ingredients

6 tablespoons 100% cocoa powder

60g (2 ½ oz) plain flour

200g (7oz) caster sugar

2 tablespoons vegetable or nut oil

1 teaspoon vanilla extract

125g (4oz) pitted dates, pureed in a blender

2 eggs

Pinch of salt

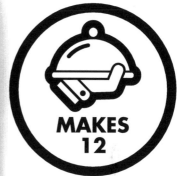

MAKES 12

Method

Grease and line a square cake tin. Place the cocoa power, flour, sugar and salt in a bowl. Stir in the dates, eggs, oil and vanilla extract. Mix until smooth. Pour the mixture into the cake tin. Bake in the oven at 180C/350F for 30 minutes. Check if it's cooked by inserting a skewer which should come out clean. Allow to cool and cut into squares.

Strawberry & Banana Milk Shake

Ingredients

200ml (7fl oz) almond milk
1 cup fresh strawberries, stalks removed
1/2 a banana

SERVES
1

Method

Place all the ingredients into a blender and blitz until smooth

Fruit Kebabs With Strawberry & Mint Dip

Ingredients

150g (5oz) grapes
1 melon, cut into cubes
400g (14oz) strawberries
4 mint leaves

Juice of 1/2 lime
1 tablespoon olive oil
2 tablespoons lemon juice

SERVES
4

Method

Place 100g (3½ oz) of the strawberries together with the lime juice and mint leaves into a food processor and blitz until smooth. Thread the remaining fruit alternately onto the skewers. Serve along with the strawberry and mint dip.

Rice Pudding With Cinnamon & Nuts

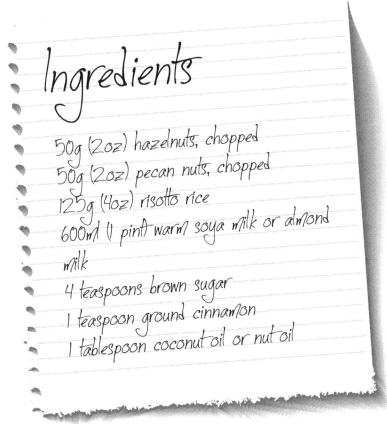

Ingredients

50g (2oz) hazelnuts, chopped
50g (2oz) pecan nuts, chopped
125g (4oz) risotto rice
600ml (1 pint) warm soya milk or almond milk
4 teaspoons brown sugar
1 teaspoon ground cinnamon
1 tablespoon coconut oil or nut oil

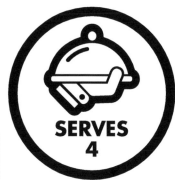

SERVES 4

Method

Heat a dry frying pan and add the nuts. Toast the nuts until lightly golden then set aside. Heat the oil in a saucepan and add the rice. Stir and cook for around 1 minute. Slowly add the warm milk to the rice, stirring continuously. Add the sugar and cinnamon and simmer gently for around 20 minutes. Serve the rice pudding into bowls. Chop the toasted nuts and sprinkle them on top of the rice pudding.

Chocolate Strawberries

Ingredients

1 punnet of strawberries, washed and stems intact
150g (5oz) dairy-free chocolate

SERVES
2

Method

Heat a saucepan containing water and place a heat-proof bowl on top. Place the chocolate in the bowl and melt the chocolate until smooth, stirring occasionally. Dip each strawberry into the chocolate and coat ¾ the way up. Place the strawberry onto a wire rack, stem side pointing down. Chill before serving.

Strawberry & Mint Granita

Ingredients

350g (12oz) strawberries
4 fresh mint leaves

SERVES
4

Method

Place the strawberries and mint leaves into a food processor and blitz until smooth. Pour into a container and freeze. Every few hours beat the mixture with a fork. Freeze until firm and granular. Remove from the freezer 10 minutes before serving. Serve into a decorative dish or glass. It's wonderfully refreshing!

Barbecued Pineapple

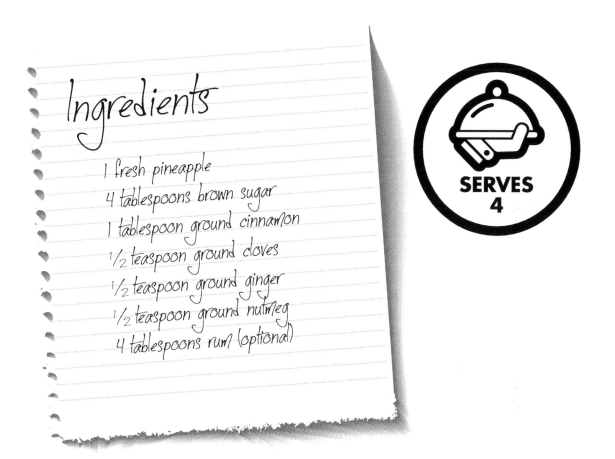

Ingredients

1 fresh pineapple
4 tablespoons brown sugar
1 tablespoon ground cinnamon
1/2 teaspoon ground cloves
1/2 teaspoon ground ginger
1/2 teaspoon ground nutmeg
4 tablespoons rum (optional)

SERVES
4

Method

Peel and core the pineapple. Cut into rings. Put the sugar, rum, ginger, nutmeg, cinnamon and cloves into a large bowl and mix together. Add the pineapple and coat it in the spice mixture. Allow to marinate for at least an hour or more if you can. Heat the barbecue to a high heat. Cook for around 7 minutes on each side until char-grilled. Serve hot with dairy-free ice cream.

Cinnamon Hot Chocolate

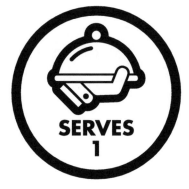

SERVES 1

Ingredients

300ml (½ pint) almond or rice milk
¼ teaspoon cinnamon
1½ teaspoons 100% cocoa powder
1 tablespoon honey, or to taste
Cocoa powder and a cinnamon stick,
to garnish

Method

Place all the ingredients, except the cinnamon stick, into a saucepan and mix well. Warm the milk, reduce the heat and simmer for 3 minutes. Whisk it really well to make it frothy. Pour into your favourite mug. Add a little extra cinnamon or honey if required. Sprinkle with cocoa powder. Place the cinnamon stick in the mug and enjoy.

Peanut Butter Hot Chocolate

Ingredients

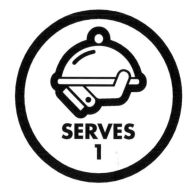

SERVES
1

200ml (7fl oz) coconut milk
100ml (3 ½ fl oz) of rice or almond milk
1 tablespoon smooth peanut butter
1 ½ teaspoons 100% cocoa powder
1 tablespoon honey, or to taste
Cocoa powder to garnish

Method

Place all the ingredients into a saucepan and mix well. Warm the milk to boiling point, reduce the heat and simmer for 1 minute. Whisk it really well to make it frothy. Pour into a mug and add a little honey if required. Sprinkle with cocoa powder. Enjoy.

SAUCES AND CONDIMENTS

Chocolate Hazelnut Spread

Ingredients

140g (4 ½ oz) hazelnuts

120ml (4fl oz) coconut milk

2 tablespoons honey

25g (1oz) 100% cocoa powder

1 teaspoon vanilla extract

¼ teaspoon salt

Method

Sprinkle the hazelnuts on a baking tray and bake at 180C/350F for 8-10 minutes. Remove any excess skins. Place the hazelnuts in a food processor and blitz until they are smooth. Add the coconut milk, honey, cocoa power, vanilla essence and salt and process until you have a smooth paste. Transfer to a jar and store in the fridge.

Guacamole

Ingredients

- 2 ripe avocados
- 1 clove garlic
- 1 red chilli pepper, finely chopped
- Juice of 1 lime
- 2 tablespoons fresh coriander leaves (cilantro), chopped

Method

Remove the stone from the avocado and scoop out the flesh. Combine all the ingredients in a bowl and mash together until smooth. Garnish with fresh coriander.

Hummus

Ingredients

- 225g (8oz) can of chickpeas (garbanzo beans), drained
- 2 cloves garlic
- Juice of 1 lemon
- 1 tablespoon olive oil
- 1 teaspoon sea salt

Method

Place all the ingredients in a blender until it is combined. Transfer the hummus into a bowl and it's ready to serve as a dip for crudities.

Avocado Salsa

Ingredients

2 ripe avocados, peeled and diced

2 large ripe tomatoes, de-seeded and chopped

6 spring onions, finely chopped

1 red chilli, de-seeded and chopped

2 handfuls coriander (cilantro) leaves

Juice of 1 lime

Extra coriander (cilantro) for garnish

Method

Combine all the ingredients in a bowl and stir. Place in a serving bowl. Sprinkle with a little coriander to garnish. Serve with fish and meat dishes or even add to a salad.

Basil Pesto

Ingredients

4 handfuls of fresh basil leaves

1 clove of garlic

40g (1 1/2 oz) pine nuts

2 tablespoons olive oil

1/4 teaspoon salt

1 teaspoon lemon juice

Method

Put all the ingredients in a blender and blitz until smooth. You can add extra olive oil to make the consistency thinner if required.

Cajun Seasoning

Ingredients

2 ½ tablespoons paprika
2 tablespoons sea salt
2 tablespoons garlic powder
1 tablespoon onion powder

1 tablespoon cayenne pepper
1 tablespoon dried oregano
1 tablespoon dried thyme

Method

Mix the ingredients together in a bowl, store in a container or jar and add this versatile seasoning to chicken, seafood, chops and steak.

Jerk Seasoning

Ingredients

2 teaspoons thyme
1 teaspoon ground allspice
1 tablespoon onion powder
½ teaspoon ground cinnamon
1 teaspoon honey

½ teaspoon ground nutmeg
1 teaspoon black pepper
1 teaspoon cayenne pepper
1 teaspoon salt

Method

Mix all of the ingredients together and store in a container. Sprinkle the seasoning onto chops, chicken or fish before cooking.

117

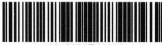

Printed in Great Britain
by Amazon